Contents

Safeguarding Patients

The Government's response
to the recommendations of the
Shipman Inquiry's fifth report and to
the recommendations of the Ayling,
Neale and Kerr/Haslam Inquiries

Presented to Parliament
by the Secretary of State for Health
by command of Her Majesty

February 2007

Cm 7015   London: the Stationery Office   £25.00

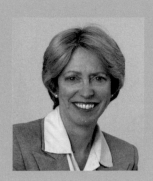

Foreword by
The Secretary of State for Health

We are rightly proud of the dedication, skill and hard work of the professionals and front-line staff who work in the National Health Service. All of us have, from time to time, entrusted our health or that of our families to health staff. In the vast majority of cases, that trust is well placed. Opinion polls repeatedly show that, of all occupations, health professionals such as doctors and nurses are the most trusted.

It is therefore all the more bewildering when that trust is betrayed. Sadly, a number of high-profile cases in recent years have reminded us that even members of caring professions can fall away from the high standards to which they are committed.

This report sets out the action which the government is taking in response to four reports relating to the abuse of trust by health professionals – the Shipman Inquiry's Fifth Report, and the reports of the Ayling, Neale and Kerr/Haslam Inquiries. The nature of the abuse differs between the four reports, but the underlying question is the same in each case: why did the NHS at the time fail to identify the risk and take the appropriate action to protect patients? The government is profoundly grateful to the chairs of the four inquiries – Dame Janet (now Lady Justice) Smith, Dame Anna Pauffley, Suzan Matthews QC and Nigel Pleming QC – and to their panels, legal teams and specialist advisors, for their meticulous work and the care with which they have sought in their recommendations to balance the need for additional safeguards with the need to avoid placing unnecessary obstacles in the way of the normal processes of patient care.

The case of Harold Shipman, the trusted GP from Hyde in Greater Manchester who murdered around 250 of his patients over a 20-year period, is well known. The Government has already set out proposals for action in relation to the recommendations of the Second Report (on the original police investigation) and the Fourth Report (on the special safeguards needed for controlled drugs) and on the proposals for reform of the coroners' system in the Third Report. Much of this action is already underway. Today we are publishing this formal response to the recommendations in the Fifth Report, relating to the monitoring and local discipline of health professionals and the handling of complaints and concerns; a White Paper *Trust, assurance and safety* with proposals for fundamental change to the regulation of health professionals in the UK; and outline proposals for change to the scrutiny of death certificates. We are also publishing an overview paper, *Learning from tragedy*, which summarises the action which the government is taking in all these separate fields.

The subjects of the other three inquiries are perhaps less well known. Neale was an obstetrician who was struck off the register in Canada for incompetent performance of surgical procedures but nevertheless managed to maintain his registration and obtain employment in the UK for several years afterwards. Ayling – a GP in Sussex – and Kerr and Haslam – consultant psychiatrists in York – were responsible over many years for the sexual abuse of female patients. These inquiries raise many similar issues to those of the Shipman Inquiry's Fifth Report – the failure to take sufficient account of complaints and concerns, the failure to join up information available in different organisations, the failure to investigate serious allegations with an appropriate degree of rigour – as well some specific issues relating to recruitment processes, maintaining appropriate boundaries between professionals and their patients, and the need for particular precautions in relation to vulnerable patients such as those suffering from mental illness.

As the Shipman Inquiry acknowledged, the NHS has made much progress since the period covered by the four inquiries in setting up general structures and processes ("clinical governance") to ensure the quality of care and to promote continuous quality improvement. If these processes had been in place, it is highly unlikely that abuses could have continued for such long periods without being detected.

Nevertheless, the government accepts that further safeguards are needed. This response sets out the action we will be taking forward. Our overriding aim is to enhance patient safety, but without placing undue obstacles in the way of patient care. We intend to do so by building on and strengthening existing clinical governance processes, following the approach to controlled drugs set out in our response to the Shipman Inquiry's Fourth Report.

There are still people who say that Shipman was unique; that it is futile to attempt to strengthen the existing safeguards, because any future individual who wanted to harm patients would evade them by using different methods; and that any additional safeguards will only have the effect of undermining the bond of trust between patient and healthcare professional and of impeding the delivery of patient care. The Government does not accept this point of view. We believe that the government's programme of action set out in this response, and in the complementary White Paper on professional regulation, will provide patients with robust safeguards against abuse, while ensuring that the vast majority of health professionals are still supported and respected as they seek to deliver the best possible care to their patients.

Executive Summary

1. This is the formal Government response to the recommendations of the Shipman Inquiry's fifth report and the reports of the Ayling, Neale and Kerr/Haslam Inquiries. It deals mainly with enhancements to the systems in place in healthcare organisations to identify, investigate and respond to actions by health professionals which could put the safety and wellbeing of patients at risk. It should be read in conjunction with the White Paper *Trust, assurance and safety: the regulation of health professionals in the 21st century*, which deals with similar issues from the perspective of professional regulation. Action arising from the two documents will be carried forward as a single, integrated work programme.

The four inquiries

2. Chapter 1 of the response summarises briefly the themes of the four inquiry reports. The details vary but the underlying issue is the same in each case: how was it possible for health professionals to continue so long to abuse – in Shipman's case, to murder – patients without anyone in authority apparently noticing, let alone taking effective action? The inquiry reports therefore deal with questions such as:

- appointment and screening processes;

- the use of routine monitoring data to detect apparent failures in professional performance;

- the "triangulation" of information from different sources;

- the use of information from complaints and from concerns expressed by health professionals;

- the systems in place in health organisations to deal with performance and behavioural issues; and

- the response of the national health professions regulators to concerns raised.

3. The reports between them contain a total of 228 recommendations, some relating to primary medical care, some to secondary care and some to special clinical settings such as mental health. The Government's response seeks where possible to generalise and to propose action that would enhance the safety of patients in all healthcare settings and for all professional groups.

The wider context

4. The crimes addressed by the four inquiries were committed many years ago, some dating back to the 1970s and 1980s. As the inquiry reports recognise, both the NHS and the context in which it operates have changed radically since then. Chapter 2 summarises some of the key developments in recent years which are relevant to the inquiry's recommendations, in particular:

- the overall quality strategy set out in *A first class service* in 1998, with explicit standards monitored by what is now the Healthcare Commission;

- recent developments in the regulation of healthcare organisations;

- the central role of clinical governance in assuring quality and promoting quality improvement;

- new approaches to handling disciplinary and performance issues in both primary and secondary care, including the role of the National Clinical Assessment Service (NCAS) to advise employers and primary care trusts (PCTs);

- the developing patient safety agenda launched by *An organisation with a memory* in 2000;

- the increasing recognition of the role of patients' experience and involvement in shaping services and in providing feedback to improve service quality;

- the movement towards a "patient-led NHS" and the wider health reform programme;

- the "better regulation" programme and the need to ensure that the burden on frontline staff is proportionate to the risks averted.

Recruitment and screening processes

5. Chapter 3 addresses the recommendations of the Neale Inquiry on recruitment and screening processes in health organisations. Guidance in this area is issued by NHS Employers, a part of the NHS Confederation, and has already been updated to meet some of the Neale recommendations. The Government:

- will consider the best way of using the new approach to regulation set out in a recent consultation paper[i] to promote best practice in this area; and

- has asked NHS Employers to ensure that future updates of its guidance take account of all the Neale Inquiry's recommendations.

Clinical governance

6. "Clinical governance" is a concept first introduced in *The new NHS: modern, dependable* in 1997 and in *A first class service* the following year. It describes both a culture and a set of processes and structures to assure quality and to commit all health staff to continuous quality improvement. These processes include as a subset the processes needed to identify poor practice or behaviour in individual health professionals, investigate complaints and concerns, and take effective action to ensure patient safety and (where possible) help the individuals to remedy their shortcomings.

7. Chapter 4 sets out the Government's belief that action to respond to the central concerns of the four inquiries should build on and strengthen existing clinical governance processes, not replace them. This is fully consistent with the approach taken by the Government to improving the

---

i *The future regulation of health and adult social care in England* (Department of Health, December 2006)

management of controlled drugs in response to the Shipman Inquiry's fourth report[ii] and with the proposed reform of procedures for scrutinising death certificates outlined in a companion paper published today[iii].

8. The Government fully accepts that more needs to be done to strengthen clinical governance processes and to embed the culture of clinical governance in every NHS organisation. Among other changes announced in this chapter, the Government

- will consider how the statutory "duty of quality" on all NHS organisations can be strengthened to underline the duty to investigate and learn from complaints and medical errors;

- will issue further guidance on the investigation of complaints and concerns, including overlapping investigations involving the police or health professions regulators;

- as part of this work, has asked the Commission for Healthcare Regulatory Excellence (CHRE) to lead a project to define the standards for local investigations so that their findings could be used by professional regulators, and to determine the thresholds at which concerns should be referred on to the regulators;

- will consider extending the role of the NCAS to provide advice to healthcare organisations for health professionals other than doctors and dentists;

- in primary care, will consider how the accountability of GPs to their PCT can be further strengthened[iv], as proposed in the Chief Medical Officer's (CMO's) review of medical regulation, including clarifying the right of access of PCTs to patients' medical records when needed in the course of an investigation; and

- will review the Performers List arrangements, including considering the Shipman Inquiry's proposal for a range of lesser sanctions as an alternative to suspending or removing primary care professionals from the list.

Complaints and concerns

9. The Government agrees that complaints (from patients or their representatives) and concerns (from fellow professionals) can provide vital information in identifying potential risks to patient safety, as well as more generally indicating how services can be improved. There have already been major developments in this area in recent years. Chapter 5 summarises recent changes and refers to the major review of the complaints systems for both health and social care launched by the Department of Health in 2006 following a commitment in the community services White Paper *Our health, our care, our say*. As part of this programme the Government:

- will shortly issue a consultation paper with proposals for a new complaints system;

- as part of this consultation will consult on possible developments of the current national standards relating to the handling of complaints in health and social care[v];

---

ii *Safer management of controlled drugs* (TSO December 2004)

iii *Learning from tragedy, keeping patients safe: overview of the government's action programme in response to the recommendations of the Shipman Inquiry* (TSO February 2007)

iv *Good doctors, safer patients* (Department of Health, July 2006)

v See for instance core standard C14 in *Standards for better health* (Department of Health, July 2004), the current standards applying to NHS healthcare organisations.

- will work with stakeholders on a set of common standards for the initial handling of complaints to ensure that, wherever patients first direct a complaint, it is speedily transferred to the most appropriate organisation;

- will, subject to consultation, amend the complaints regulations to enable patients or their representatives to make complaints about treatment in general medical practice directly to their PCT, and to require PCTs to take an overview of all such complaints even where they are handled by the practice concerned;

- is supporting complaints handlers in general practice by setting up networks for mutual support;

- will ensure that all organisations providing services to NHS patients have clear policies setting out how staff can raise concerns;

- will explore the potential role of strategic health authorities (SHAs) or PCTs in receiving concerns where the member of staff feels unable to go to their own employer; and

- will explore with professional regulators and universities how the duty on health professionals to report concerns about fellow professionals can be further emphasised, especially in undergraduate education.

Boundary transgressions and particular issues in mental health services

10. Chapter 6 considers the recommendations in the Kerr/Haslam and Ayling inquiries about the failure of health organisations to take seriously allegations of sexual assault on female patients. Since the period covered by the two inquiries there has been a growing awareness of the issue of sexual or other abuse by health professionals, thanks in no small measure to the courage of the victims in coming forward and bringing their experiences into the public domain. But further work is needed to both to develop guidance and to ensure that all staff working in the NHS are fully aware of the issues.

11. The Department has commissioned the Council of Healthcare Regulatory Excellence (CHRE) to carry out a major exercise which will, among other things:

- develop detailed and comprehensive guidance for health professionals and their regulators on the proper boundaries which professionals should maintain between themselves and their patients;

- develop guidance for NHS and other healthcare employers on how to prevent, detect and investigate boundary violations; and

- develop a common approach to educational standards on boundary issues for adoption into training programmes for professionals.

12. Patients in mental health settings are particular vulnerable to potential boundary violations. Chapter 7 discusses the recommendations relating to this particular group of patients in the Kerr/Haslam report. In general, the Government believes that the principles of clinical governance which apply in other settings are equally relevant to mental health, but agrees that special attention may be needed to be given to issues such as:

- the use of information disclosed in the therapeutic setting;

- advocacy support for patients wishing to make a complaint; and

- training in mental health issues for health professionals.

The Government will discuss further with stakeholders and issue further guidance as needed.

Information

13. All four inquiries stress the key role of information in identifying potential problems of professional behaviour or competence and alerting healthcare organisations to the need to take action to protect patients. Often, relevant information is held by different organisations or different parts of one organisation, and it is only by "triangulating" this information that the true extent of problems can be revealed. At the same time, sharing information between organisations, especially "soft" information such as unsubstantiated complaints or concerns, raises difficult issues about confidentiality and the human rights of individual professionals.

14. Chapter 8 reviews the recommendations in this area from the four inquiries and from *Good doctors, safer patients*. The Government will:

- issue or commission guidance on the content of files kept by healthcare organisations about health professionals employed by or in contract with them and about the circumstances in which such information can be shared with other organisations;

- discuss with stakeholders the possibility of extending, to performance issues more generally, the concept in the 2006 Health Act[vi] of a statutory duty to share information where needed to protect the public;

- progress, with the Royal College of General Practitioners (RCGP) and other stakeholders, work on indicators of the quality of services provided by primary care practices ("practice profiling"), including the use of prescribing indicators and information on mortality; and

- discuss further the proposal from the Shipman Inquiry that GPs should be required to disclose all clinical negligence claims to their PCT.

15. In addition, as announced in *Trust, assurance and safety*, the Government has accepted the recommendations in the CMO's review that the GMC register should become the main source of information on doctors' registration status and on any disciplinary action, including "recorded concerns" (a formal note of a concern over professional conduct or competency which the doctor has accepted but is not regarded as significant enough to require referral to the GMC's central fitness to practise proceedings). There will be "tiered" access to this information, with some parts of the information base generally available and other parts available only to NHS and other accredited healthcare employers.

Taking the action forward

16. As already noted, the action stemming from this document and from *Trust, assurance and safety* should be seen as a single programme of action to ensure patient safety, and to reassure the public that the NHS has learnt from the lessons of the Shipman and other high-profile cases. Although the broad thrust is clear, many issues of detail remain which the Department of Health

---

vi See Health Act 2006 section 18. At present this statutory duty to collaborate by sharing information and agreeing appropriate joint action is limited to issues related to the abuse or diversion of controlled drugs, responding to concerns set out in the Shipman Inquiry's fourth report.

will need to discuss with patient, NHS, and professional groups and with the health professions regulators. The Department will:

- in due course publish an integrated action plan setting out a timetable for all the action envisaged in the two documents; and

- establish a national advisory group with all relevant stakeholders to advise the Department on implementation.

Chapter 1
Introduction

The fifth report: lessons learnt

1.1 The Shipman Inquiry's fifth report, *Safeguarding patients: lessons from the past, proposals for the future*[1], was published in December 2004. It is the last of three reports which between them seek to answer the questions: how was it possible for Harold Shipman to continue to murder patients for so many years without detection; and what needs to be done to protect patients in the future?

1.2 Whereas the third report[2] examines the certification and investigation of deaths and the failure of the system then current to draw attention to Shipman's misdeeds, and the fourth report[3] focuses on weaknesses in the systems for safeguarding the use of controlled drugs, the fifth report looks more generally at the arrangements for safeguarding patients from incompetent or aberrant performance by health professionals. In particular, the fifth report reviews:

- the arrangements in NHS primary care for **monitoring the standards of care** of health professionals and for taking action to protect patients where there is cause for concern;

- the handling of **complaints** from patients and **expressions of concern** from fellow professionals;

- the developing proposals from the General Medical Council (GMC) for a system for periodic **revalidation** of doctors' licence to practise; and

- the GMC's procedures for dealing with doctors whose **fitness to practise** has been called into question.

1.3 The inquiry recognised that all these systems, as well as the general context in which they are operating, are in a state of change. It therefore took pains to consider not only what systems were operating at the time of Shipman's crimes but also the extent to which recent developments might have provided better safeguards. In some aspects, the fifth report is broadly supportive of current developments, and its recommendations are intended to reinforce and guide what is already in progress. In other aspects – in particular, those relating to revalidation and to the GMC's fitness to practise procedures – the report is more critical of current developments and sets out its alternative views on how patients should be best protected.

1.4 The report's recommendations, for understandable reasons, focus primarily on identifying and dealing with the extremes of unacceptable professional behaviour. However, as the inquiry fully recognised, the vast majority of health professionals are committed to providing good care for their patients. The inquiry therefore emphasised that their recommendations are intended to work alongside the more general systems and processes, collectively known as clinical governance, through which the NHS seeks to promote high standards of clinical care.

1.5 Although the inquiry's terms of reference were limited to primary care, and the focus is therefore on the monitoring and assessment of primary care doctors (general practitioners), the inquiry recognised that much of its analysis has implications for health professionals more generally and for secondary as well as primary care settings.

The Ayling, Neale and Kerr/Haslam Inquiries

1.6 At more or less the same time as the Shipman Inquiry, three other inquiries published their findings, the inquiries into the cases of Clifford Ayling[4], Richard Neale[5], and William Kerr and Michael Haslam[6] (see Annex A for their terms of reference). Although each of these has its particular features, there is a common thread running through all four inquiries: the failure of those in positions of authority in the NHS or in the regulators to detect signs of unacceptable or incompetent professional behaviour and to take effective and timely action to protect patients. It therefore makes sense to consider the common aspects of all four sets of recommendations together, as indeed the Kerr/Haslam inquiry suggests[7]. In doing so, we fully recognise the important contribution made by each inquiry and the need to address the particular issues and recommendations of each.

Taking forward the recommendations

1.7 Shortly after publication of the fifth report, the then Secretary of State for Health announced that he had asked Professor Sir Liam Donaldson, the Chief Medical Officer (CMO), to carry out a review of some aspects of medical regulation and to give his personal advice to ministers on his conclusions. Subsequently, the Government announced a parallel review of regulation of the non-medical professions to be carried out by Andrew Foster, Director of Human Resources of the Department of Health. The terms of reference of the two reviews are at Annex B.

1.8 The conclusions of the two reviews were published in July 2006[8,9] and were followed by a three-month consultation, which ended in November. In parallel with this formal response to the recommendations of the four inquiries, the Government is today publishing a White Paper *Trust, assurance and safety – the regulation of health professionals in the 21st century*[10], setting out its decisions on the future arrangements for the regulation of the health professions. Many of the detailed recommendations in the Shipman Inquiry's fifth report are either addressed directly in *Trust, assurance and safety* or will fall to the regulators for the individual professions to take forward in the light of the general framework which it sets out.

1.9 This response therefore addresses the complementary issues raised by the Shipman Inquiry's fifth report and by the Ayling, Neale and Kerr/Haslam inquiries (the "three inquiries"). It describes the context in which implementation will take place in England[vii], including the implications of the policies summarised in *Creating a patient-led NHS*[11] and subsequent publications[12], and sets out the Department's broad approach to implementation. In particular, the response draws attention to the major developments which have taken place in the NHS in recent years in the fields of quality and patient safety; and suggests that

- the best way of protecting patients is to build on and strengthen the existing arrangements for promoting the quality of clinical care, collectively known as clinical governance;

- the vast majority of health professionals are already giving high-quality care to their patients; for them, clinical governance arrangements are intended to provide support, encouragement and time for reflection on their clinical practice; and

vii Regulation of certain of the professions is a reserved matter for the UK Parliament. Local implementation in Scotland, Wales and Northern Ireland, and regulation of the remaining professions, will be determined by the respective administrations, although the broad approach is likely to be similar. References to primary care trusts (PCTs) should be understood as applying where appropriate to the equivalent bodies in the other parts of the United Kingdom.

- a very small minority exhibit behaviour or clinical performance which puts patients at risk. Clinical governance needs to be sufficiently robust to maximise the chance of identifying these clinicians so that prompt action can be taken to protect patients. But no system can give an absolute guarantee of safety, especially (as the Shipman Inquiry fully recognised) when faced with an individual as devious and malign as Shipman.

1.10 The response then goes on to

- set out in full the action which the Department proposes to take to strengthen the overall capability of the NHS to deal with the common challenges described in the four inquiries;

- describe the action proposed or already under way to address the specific areas addressed by the Ayling, Neale and Kerr/Haslam inquiries, and in particular the issues of sexualised behaviour (Ayling and Kerr/Haslam), special protection for mental health patients (Kerr/Haslam) and recruitment processes (Neale); and

- consider the implications for all healthcare professions, and for secondary as well as primary care, within a general clinical governance framework applicable in all settings.

Separate annexes to the response (Annexes C to F) show in turn for each of the inquiry reports how each recommendation is being progressed, including cross-references as appropriate to *Trust, assurance and safety*.

1.11 The final section of the response summarises the action which the Department already has in hand or is proposing to strengthen existing safeguards. Following consultation with stakeholders on details of the proposed actions, the Department will publish an integrated action plan, covering both the reform of professional regulation and the other action in this response, and setting out a more detailed timetable for the proposed legislative and regulatory changes and for the associated guidance to the NHS.

Overview of the Government's response to the Shipman Inquiry

1.12 In parallel with this response, the Government is publishing *Learning from tragedy – keeping patients safe*[13], a summary of all the action in hand or proposed to take forward the recommendations of the Shipman Inquiry. This paper

- gives a broad overview of the challenges posed by the Shipman case, in particular the failure of the systems then in place, over such a long period, to detect his crimes and to respond to the signals that were available; and

- shows how action across four government departments – and covering the disparate fields of death certification, the coroners' system, management of controlled drugs, management of professional performance and professional regulation – together make up a coherent programme of action to deal with these challenges and to protect patients and the general public in the future.

As the Shipman Inquiry recognised, it will never be possible to give complete protection against the actions of a criminal as devious and sophisticated as a Shipman. The Government however believes that the actions it is undertaking in these various fields will act as an effective deterrent, and will make it highly unlikely that any future criminal could continue for long without detection.

Chapter 2
The Wider Context

Quality standards and the regulation of healthcare organisations

2.1 The 1998 consultation paper *A first class service*[14] set out a broad strategy for promoting clinical quality in the NHS. The strategy comprises three interlocking components:

- explicit **standards** describing the quality of care which patients can expect to receive;

- assurance of, and continuous improvement in, the systems and processes for **local delivery** of healthcare through clinical governance; and

- national **monitoring** of performance in relation to the standards.

2.2 Quality standards relating to individual services or interventions are published in guidance documents from the National Institute for Health and Clinical Excellence (NICE) and in National Service Frameworks. Generic quality standards for the NHS ("Standards for better health") were set out in *National standards, local action*[15] in seven "domains", including patient safety, clinical effectiveness and governance (see below). Within each domain, the standards are divided into **core standards** which all NHS organisations are expected to achieve, and **developmental standards** which are to be achieved over a period and provide a framework for continuous improvement in quality.

2.3 Responsibility for the assessment of NHS primary care trusts (PCTs) and specialist services rests with the Healthcare Commission, whose remit largely derives from the recommendations of the Bristol Royal Infirmary Inquiry[16]. Each year the Healthcare Commission publishes its assessment of the performance of all NHS organisations against each of the standards, leading to an overall rating based on the balance of performance across all seven domains.

2.4 Healthcare providers in the independent and voluntary sectors are assessed against regulations issued under the Care Standards Act 2000 and underpinned by a different set of standards, the National Minimum Standards[17]; compliance with these regulations is a precondition of registration by the Healthcare Commission (for hospitals and clinics) or by the Commission for Social Care Inspection (for care homes). The Department intends in the near future to amend the regulations and *National Minimum Standards* to align them with the *Standards for better health*, so that all healthcare organisations can be assessed on the same basis.

2.5 More fundamental changes to the regulation of healthcare organisations were recently announced in *The future regulation of health and adult social care in England*[18]. This document proposes that, with effect from 2009-10, all healthcare providers in secondary care, including NHS providers, should be included within an integrated registration regime and assessed against national standards of quality and safety. Organisations failing to give assurance that they are meeting these standards would need to take urgent remedial action and could, in the last resort, face losing registration in relation to the services in question. The document also seeks views on how these principles might be applied to primary medical care. The Department will be consulting later in 2007 on the national standards needed to underpin registration and on their relation to the existing core standards; and on the application of these principles to providers of non-medical primary care.

Clinical governance

2.6 The concept of "clinical governance" was first introduced in *The new NHS – modern, dependable*[19] and described more fully in *A first class service: quality in the new NHS* and later publications[20]. It describes both an overall approach to improving the quality of care and a set of specific systems processes. At the most general level, clinical governance asserts that healthcare organisations have a **corporate responsibility**, over and above the responsibility of **individual** health professionals working in the organisation, to provide safe and high quality care and to strive for continuous quality improvement. Clinical governance seeks to embed the culture and systems needed to promote quality improvement and patient safety into the everyday routines of every clinical team. The systems, processes and behaviours underlying clinical governance include

- effective leadership at all levels;

- effective multi-disciplinary team working;

- formal processes for the assessment and uptake of new healthcare technologies and for the implementation of new guidance from NICE and National Service Frameworks;

- participation of all clinicians in multi-disciplinary clinical audit and continuous professional development;

- benchmarking of clinical quality indicators against best national or international practice;

- provision of information to patients about their condition and treatment options to enable informed patient choice;

- proactive sampling of patient and user feedback on the quality of the services provided;

- meaningful engagement of patients, carers and the general public in the development of services;

- proactive risk assessment and management of clinical processes and the environment in which care is delivered;

- learning from patients' complaints and expressions of concern from professionals;

- systematic learning through root cause analysis of patient safety incidents (including significant "near misses") to enable local learning;

- full participation in the National Patient Safety Agency's National Learning and Reporting System (see para 2.14 below); and

- robust and transparent processes for identifying and investigating concerns over the performance or behaviour of individual clinicians and managers, and taking appropriate action (with the health professions regulators as appropriate) to protect patients and the wider public.

2.7 All general medical practices, community pharmacies and specialist healthcare providers in the NHS are required to appoint a clinical governance lead of appropriate seniority to set up these processes and to ensure that they are effective. In addition, in primary care, PCTs are required to appoint a clinical governance lead (usually a local GP) with specific responsibility for

- promoting the understanding and uptake of clinical governance concepts by primary care practices, community pharmacies and other providers in contract with the PCT;

- enabling the sharing of learning from incidents and best practice across the whole health community; and

- setting up PCT-wide systems for monitoring clinical quality through indicators such as prescribing indicators.

PCTs are also required to ensure that all NHS dental practices have robust clinical governance arrangements.

Handling performance issues

Primary care: list management

2.8 Although PCTs do not (in general) have a conventional employer-employee relationship with frontline primary care staff, they do have a range of powers available to protect patients in cases where the competence or behaviour of individual practitioners could put patients at risk, the **list management** powers. These were introduced in 2001[22] in response to a series of high profile cases which drew attention to the inadequacy of existing procedures. In developing the new procedures, the Department sought to ensure that:

- all doctors performing primary care services featured on a list of practitioners held by the PCT; and

- PCTs could suspend doctors promptly while investigating concerns about their practice.

These powers enable PCTs to act swiftly and decisively to avert harm to patients, while being fair to the doctor whose livelihood could be at stake. The procedures allow the PCT to consider the case against the doctor and give the doctor the opportunity to respond. There is a right of appeal to the Family Health Services Appeal Authority (FHSAA). These arrangements will be reviewed in the course of 2007 in the light of the other changes to the regulatory system (see para 4.35 below).

Secondary care

2.9 New disciplinary processes were set out in 2005 in *Maintaining high professional standards in the modern NHS*[23]. This new framework applies the same locally based procedures to all employees of NHS organisations in England, including doctors and dentists, and removes the previous distinction between personal and professional misconduct. NHS employers are also, like other employers, bound by the Employment Acts and are required to follow good practice guidance from the Advisory, Conciliation and Arbitration Service[24].

2.10 Some of the key features of the new framework are as follows:

- *investigation*: the guidance sets out clear responsibilities for the investigation of concerns, and for the seniority of the investigator. Trusts are encouraged to ensure that several clinical managers are trained in investigation techniques to enable them to undertake this role when required;

- *separation of investigation and decision-making*: in line with the principles of natural justice, the guidance requires a clear separation between those who investigate concerns and allegations (in order to establish the facts) and those who subsequently decide what action is needed. The guidance recommends that final decisions are taken by a subcommittee of the trust board chaired by a senior executive, eg the Medical Director;

- *the role of remediation*: employers are encouraged to consider the possibility of remediation where this would not put patient safety at risk. In cases involving the performance of doctors and dentists, employers are required to seek the advice of the National Clinical Assessment Service (see next section);

- *less reliance on suspension*: the new procedures are explicitly designed to reduce the reliance on lengthy periods of exclusion from work.

The National Clinical Assessment Service

2.11 Where a clinician's performance gives cause for concern, employers and PCTs will often need expert advice in deciding what action is needed, for instance whether the apparent deficiency can be relatively easily corrected or whether there is a more deep-seated problem. The 1999 consultation document *Supporting doctors, protecting patients*[25] introduced the concept of "clinical assessment" and led to the setting up of an expert resource, the National Clinical Assessment Authority (now the National Clinical Assessment Service (NCAS) of the National Patient Safety Agency).

2.12 NCAS provides general guidance to the NHS and advice to employers and PCTs on the handling of individual cases involving doctors and dentists. National policies[26] require NHS employers to seek NCAS advice at all key stages of investigations and disciplinary procedures. NCAS will also, if invited, carry out a full assessment of the clinician's performance. The role of NCAS is to provide advice and support throughout the process, but final responsibility for action rests with the employer or PCT.

Patient safety

2.13 Patient safety can be regarded as a fundamental component of clinical quality, but over recent years it has received much attention in its own right. The current patient safety strategy in the NHS derives from the 2000 publication of *An organisation with a memory*[27] following a careful study which looked at approaches to safety both in other high-risk industries and internationally. The key insights from this study are that

- clinical error usually results from human error provoked by underlying system weaknesses;

- the NHS has traditionally been weak in learning collectively from errors – some serious clinical errors are repeated time and time again in different parts of the NHS;

- promoting active learning from mistakes requires

  - moving from a "blame culture" to a "safety culture" in which clinical staff are encouraged to report errors and near misses so that learning can take place; and

  - systematic processes for reporting and analysing errors, establishing the underlying causes, and ensuring that lessons are put into practice.

2.14 *Building a safer NHS for patients*[28] set out a plan for implementing the recommendations of *An organisation with a memory*. The key elements were

- setting up a new "national reporting and learning system" (NRLS) for learning from adverse events;

- building expertise in the NHS in root cause analysis;

- promoting a culture of incident reporting and patient safety in NHS organisations; and

- ensuring a more consistent approach to the commissioning of investigations to respond to failures of whole services or major systems weaknesses.

A new National Patient Safety Agency (NPSA) was set up to oversee the new national learning system, to analyse trends and to issue guidance on safety solutions to address the most serious problems identified by the system.

2.15 The National Audit Office (NAO) has recently reported on the implementation of these policies[29]. Key findings are that NHS organisations have made good progress in developing a "no blame" culture, but that levels of reporting to the NRLS are variable and especially low in primary care.

2.16 The Department accepts that more needs to be done to establish a true patient safety culture and to strengthen both reporting to the NRLS and the use made of the NRLS data. The Healthcare Commission is from this year (2006-07) assessing performance against the developmental standards in the patient safety domain, and this will help to promote the further development of a patient safety culture throughout the NHS. In addition, the Department recently invited Pauline Philip, programme lead for patient safety at the World Health Organisation, and Sir Ian Carruthers, former acting Chief Executive for the NHS, to review the implementation of patient safety arrangements in the NHS. Their report was published in December 2006[30]. Key recommendations include

- establishment of a high-level National Patient Safety Forum jointly chaired by the CMO and the NHS Chief Executive;

- development of patient safety action teams (PSATs), hosted by strategic health authorities, to support the local delivery of the patient safety agenda; and

- NHS organisations to have prime responsibility for investigating safety incidents but with access to a specialist investigator based in the local PSAT.

Patient experience and patient involvement

2.17 The last 20 or so years have seen a major shift in attitudes. There is an increasing recognition that patients should be seen not as "passive" recipients of healthcare interventions chosen and delivered by health professionals, but as active participants with their own values and beliefs. Patients and carers therefore have a vital role to play both in helping to define what counts as "quality" in healthcare – for instance, the importance of dignity and respect – and in drawing attention to unacceptable standards of care.

2.18 Among the many developments in this field some of the more significant are

- an increasing recognition of the importance of **information** to enable patients to make informed choices in dialogue with clinicians and to take better control of their own health – see for instance the Department's three-year information strategy *Better information, better choices, better health*[31];

- the development and roll-out of **expert patient programmes**[32] for patients with long-term conditions such as asthma and diabetes to help them to take active control of their own treatment;

- a systematic approach to the use of information from patient satisfaction surveys, involving all hospital trusts and administered by the Healthcare Commission, to assess and improve services – over one million patients have taken part in the surveys so far;

- a specific duty on all organisations[33] to involve patients and the general public in the planning and development of services;

- the development of Patient Liaison Services (PALS) and the Independent Complaints Advocacy Service (ICAS) to help patients, their carers and families to navigate services, find solutions when things go wrong and (where necessary) raise a formal complaint about services. Both these services act as a powerful lever for change by providing feedback and highlighting best practice;

- the provision of direct mechanisms to enable patients to report patient safety episodes directly to the NPSA and adverse drug reactions to the Medicines and Healthcare products Regulatory Agency (MHRA);

- the recent consultation document *A stronger local voice*[34] which proposes the establishment of Local Involvement Networks (LINks) to promote public and community influence in health and social care. Further details are given in the Government's response following consultation[35]; and

- the provisions in the NHS Redress Act 2006 for financial recompense to those who suffer as a result of avoidable errors in the NHS[36]. This places the emphasis on putting things right for patients as a matter of course, provides an alternative to litigation, and will contribute to the culture of learning in the NHS.

Towards a "patient-led NHS"

2.19 Recent years have seen a gradual evolution of NHS structures away from a top-down model driven by targets set by the Department of Health and towards a more devolved model in which decisions are taken by frontline staff in dialogue with patients and carers, within a framework of incentives to promote high-quality services. The rationale of this evolution was set out in 2005 in *Creating a patient-led NHS* and in the subsequent *Commissioning a patient-led NHS*, and has been more recently restated in *Health reform in England: update and next steps*[37]. Key points are

- more choice and a stronger voice for patients;

- strengthened commissioning, especially in health sectors where choice of provider is impracticable or less likely to be a major driver of quality;

- involvement of primary care practices in commissioning ("practice-based commissioning" or PBC), with PBC consortia holding notional budgets and advising PCTs on commissioning decisions, including service redesign;

- a greater variety of providers, including independent and voluntary sector providers;

- incentives which reward quality, responsiveness and value for money; and

- a unified and proportionate approach to regulation of individual healthcare organisations to ensure national standards of safety and quality.

2.20 The specific application of these principles in community care settings were set out, following an extensive consultation, in the White Paper *Our health, our care, our say*[38] published in January 2006. Among other policy proposals the White Paper

- calls for a closer alignment of health and social care services, with the aim of moving towards an integrated assessment of the performance of health economies and local authorities in which the quality of services will increasingly be judged by their outcomes for service users;

- proposes the movement of specialist services to community settings, where this can be done without detriment to quality and patient safety; and

- calls for a greater emphasis on health promotion and preventative care.

A recent report by the National Director for Primary Care, *Keeping it personal*, underlines the crucial contribution which primary care services can make.[39]

2.21 All these proposals will have significant implications for the way in which healthcare organisations, in particular PCTs, plan and commission their services and ensure the quality and safety of the care provided.

Better regulation

2.22 In the longer term, patient choice – supported by the principle under which financial flows follow the patient ("payment by results") – should be an effective lever for promoting those aspects of quality which patients can readily assess for themselves, such as convenience and dignity. However, patients can only exercise their choice effectively if they have access to reliable information about different providers, on the basis of objective assessments of processes and performance against agreed national standards. And patients will rightly expect that health professionals are fit to practise and that healthcare organisations meet essential standards of safety and clinical effectiveness, so that they can choose securely on the basis of the dimensions of quality which they can more easily judge for themselves.

2.23 There will therefore continue to be an important role for the regulation both of provider organisations and of individual health professionals. However, there has been an increasing recognition in recent years of the potential impact of regulation – not merely the direct costs of the regulator itself, but also the indirect costs in both time and money falling on the organisations or individuals being regulated. Regulation therefore needs

- to be **proportionate** to the risks of harm in the absence of regulation;

- to seek to **minimise the cost of regulation** by use of appropriate instruments such as the use of self-assessment forms instead of physical inspection visits, and by adopting an educational rather than a punitive approach where possible; and

- to be **consistent and joined up**, with different regulators working together to minimise the impact on those being regulated.

These principles were set out in the 1997 guidance from the Better Regulation Task Force *Principles of good regulation*[40] and have been powerfully reinforced in the recent report of the Hampton review[41]. The Government's proposals for the future direction of both professional regulation (as set out in *Trust, assurance and safety*) and the regulation of healthcare organisations (as set out in *The future regulation of health and adult social care in England*) are fully informed by these principles.

Chapter 3
Recruitment and Screening Processes

3.1 Deficiencies in recruitment and screening processes were not a major factor in Shipman's career. When being interviewed for his first partnership as a GP, Shipman did not conceal his previous conviction for drug offences but succeeded in convincing his future partners – as he had already convinced the GMC – that he had put the problem behind him[42]. It is therefore unlikely that any pre-recruitment screening processes would have affected the outcome.

3.2 Failures to apply proper screening processes were however a major factor in the story of Richard Neale, a consultant obstetrician who managed to retain registration with the GMC and gain appointment as a consultant in England despite having been struck off the medical register in Canada for incompetent operations. There were similar issues in the case of Beverley Allitt, a paediatric nurse who was convicted in 1993 of the murder of four children under her care at Grantham and Kesteven Hospital in Lincolnshire.

3.3 If similar tragedies are not to be repeated, all NHS organisations will need to adopt systematic processes for screening the qualifications of health professionals applying for positions. These processes should include:

- a careful scrutiny of the applicant's curriculum vitae to check for unexplained gaps in the record;

- confidential enquiries of previous employers to establish whether there was anything unusual in the previous history – this will be easier once the proposals in *Good doctors, safer patients* for "GMC affiliates" and "recorded concerns" have been implemented (see para 4.11 below); and

- a direct check of the applicant's status on the register of their professional regulator, and on any other professional qualifications claimed.

Similarly the health professions regulators should make direct checks of the claims of doctors who apply for registration in the United Kingdom on the basis of claimed experience in other countries. As the Electronic Staff Record[43] is rolled out across NHS secondary care providers in England, the checking of such "credentialing" information for existing NHS staff will be increasingly automated.

3.4 NHS Employers is already working with NHS organisations to ensure that they are aware of and applying current best practice in these areas, and published its latest guidance in January 2007[44]. The national model contract, issued as part of the 2007-08 Operating Framework[45], already requires providers to exercise an appropriate degree of "skill and care, diligence, prudence and foresight" in this regard. More generally, **the Government will consider how the new framework for regulation of all healthcare organisations** (see para 2.5) **can best reinforce this requirement**.

3.5 The rest of this chapter considers the recommendations of the Neale Inquiry in this area.

Recruitment of new staff

Recruitment processes

> Neale Inquiry recommendation 1: The Secretary of State for Health should consider setting up a new body, or expanding the power of an existing body such as the Council for Healthcare Regulatory Excellence (CHRE), to take an overarching view of all aspects of the rules governing the appointment and employment of doctors. This body should have necessary powers of investigation in the wider interests of patient safety, ensuring a robust and consistent approach to individual concerns that may arise in the future.

3.6 Guidance to the NHS on good employment practice falls within the remit of NHS Employers, a part of the NHS Confederation, and the Government considers that it would confuse NHS organisations, and detract from the safety of patients, to set up a further body for this purpose.

> Neale Inquiry recommendation 7: Clear roles should be established for all those on an interview panel and full note of proceedings should be taken and retained.
>
> Recommendation 8: All previous contacts between applicant and interviewers should be disclosed and recorded.
>
> Recommendation 9: Any undisclosed championing of applicants should be disclosed and recorded.
>
> Recommendation 10: The application form should contain a declaration that all information is correct to the best of the applicant's knowledge and belief and any matter, professional or personal unresolved or pending, that might undermine the applicant's standing, or cause embarrassment to the NHS, should be declared by a confidential side letter to the chairman. The penalty for failure to disclose such information should be summary dismissal.

3.7 The Government agrees that all these recommendations represent good practice; most are already covered in standing guidance to the NHS. **The Government will invite NHS Employers to ensure that they are fully covered in future updates of this guidance**.

Checks by employers

> Neale Inquiry recommendation 3: The contents of the model declaration forms referred to in HSC2002/08 should be made mandatory in the NHS.
>
> Recommendation 4: For all doctor appointments made directly from overseas, regardless of where they qualified, employing authorities should check with the issuing body the recommended applicant's primary and postgraduate qualifications and confirm fitness to practise.

3.8 HSC2002/08 has been superseded by more recent guidance updated in January 2007 (see para 3.4). As with other aspects of recruitment, we will consider how the new regulatory framework can best be used to promote adoption of best practice in relation to these model declaration forms.

3.9 Issues relating to the registration in the United Kingdom of doctors qualified in other countries are covered in *Trust, assurance and safety* at paras 5.14-20. The Government considers that it is for the health professions regulators to check the primary qualification of health professionals appointed from overseas and any postgraduate qualifications to be entered on the specialist register. The Government agrees that NHS organisations should check other postgraduate qualifications **and will ask NHS Employers to ensure this is reflected in guidance**, taking into account the initiative described in Chapter 6 of *Trust, assurance and safety* to promote closer cooperation between employers and regulators when health professionals enter employment in the UK for the first time.

References

Neale Inquiry recommendation 12: The Panel Chairman should be responsible for ensuring that referees are contacted by telephone and content of the references should be confirmed at or around the time of appointment.

Recommendation 14: Employing authorities/medical colleagues should not give a reference which is capable of being misleading by omission.

Kerr/Haslam Inquiry p24: One of the referees in any job application should be the consultant who conducts the applicant's appraisal, their Clinical Director, or their Medical Director.

p25: When appointments to the NHS are considered, references should be obtained from the three most recent employers and those references should be properly checked.

3.10 Existing GMC and NHS guidance already covers the ethical responsibility on health professionals to provide, and interviewing panels to look for, objective and transparent references; **the Government will invite the Council for Healthcare Regulatory Excellence (CHRE) to ensure that there is similar guidance for the other healthcare professions**. The Government agrees that panel chairmen should always be alert to the possibility of misleading references, including references from a much earlier part of the candidate's career, and **will ask NHS Employers to consider how this principle could be reflected in updated guidance**.

Security of tenure for NHS consultants

Neale Inquiry recommendation 2: Security of tenure for NHS consultants with a protective appeal procedure to the Secretary of State should be abolished.

3.11 The "para 190" right of appeal to the Secretary of State was abolished in 2005 and replaced by the new disciplinary processes set out in *Maintaining high professional standards in the modern NHS* (see para 2.9).

Previous convictions

Neale Inquiry recommendation 11: The NHS should give consideration to instruct employers to include a condition that clinical employees must declare any police cautions or convictions to the employer as they arise after the commencement of their employment.

3.12 The January 2007 update of the guidance from NHS Employers referred to above advises all NHS employers to include such a condition in contracts of employment. All health professionals are in addition under an ethical obligation to report cautions and convictions to their professional regulator, following a similar recommendation of the Shipman Inquiry's fourth report[46].

Neale Inquiry recommendation 13: The police check should include convictions, cautions and entries on the Sex Offenders Register.

3.13 Since February 2005 it has been mandatory for all NHS employers to arrange for checks at the Criminal Records Bureau (CRB) for all relevant NHS staff. The standard disclosure from the CRB shows current and spent convictions, cautions, reprimands and warnings held on the Police National Computer.

Application to primary care practitioners

3.14 In primary medical care, responsibility for ensuring that new practitioners are suitable to provide services is shared between the PCT, the individual doctor and the practice. Under these arrangements

- there is a statutory requirement under the Performers List regulations (see para 2.8) for doctors to provide a comprehensive career history, including an enhanced criminal record certificate, to the PCT before they can perform primary medical care services;

- the practice has a contractual requirement to take up two clinical references relating to recent posts before employing or engaging a health professional to perform medical services.

Similarly PCTs are required to undertaken CRB checks for dentists applying to join Performers Lists, and we intend to apply comparable arrangements for providers of primary care ophthalmic services when the provisions of the Health Act 2006 are brought into force.

Chapter 4
Clinical Governance

4.1 As already noted in Chapter 2, one of the aims of clinical governance is to ensure the safety and quality of health services by, among other things, establishing robust processes to identify and deal with poor performance by individual clinicians or clinical teams.

4.2 The Shipman Inquiry's fifth report devotes two of its chapters to reviewing arrangements for PCTs' oversight of GPs (Chapter 5) and to the development of clinical governance in primary care (Chapter 12). The broad conclusions can be summarised as follows:

- PCTs now have more information than in the 1990s on doctors whose performance may pose risks to patient safety, and more powers for protecting patients;

- there are however still some serious gaps in the available information, for instance on the details of complaints against practitioners;

- there is still widespread resistance among GPs to the idea that their clinical performance should be "managed" by PCTs;

- clinical governance potentially offers an effective means both to detect poorly performing GPs, and to help those already performing satisfactorily to do even better. However, to achieve these objectives PCTs will need much more objective information on the performance of individual doctors (not just on practices);

- PCTs are small and relatively new organisations and in many cases are struggling to fulfil their various roles;

- clinical governance is not yet fully "embedded" in primary care; clinical governance leads should be given a higher profile, better training and clearer powers.

4.3 The Department welcomes the inquiry's endorsement of the central importance of clinical governance both to improve the quality of NHS services generally and to help identify, and deal with, unacceptable performance. As the Government's response to the inquiry's fourth report[47] made clear, we believe that the key to better protection for patients is to work with the grain of existing NHS clinical governance processes rather than to replace or supplement them with something different. In this context, the key elements of clinical governance are

- embedding a learning culture in which concerns can be openly reported and addressed and appropriate action taken;

- encouraging all clinicians to take part in clinical audit and root cause analysis of adverse events so that any problems are picked up by them and their peers at the earliest possible stage;

- monitoring routine information sources (eg prescribing information, appraisals) and ad hoc sources of information (complaints, expressions of concern) in order to identify professionals whose performance or conduct could pose a threat to patient safety;

- ensuring that these concerns are investigated speedily, objectively and professionally in order to establish the facts; and

- operating fair and transparent processes to determine what action (if any) is needed to protect patients and, where possible, to help the health professional to return to acceptable standards of performance.

(It should be emphasised that clinical governance, as a set of processes and behaviours to promote excellence in healthcare, goes much wider than this; the list above focuses solely on the subset of processes required to identify and deal with potential poor performance.)

4.4 We accept the conclusion of the Shipman Inquiry that the implementation of clinical governance has been variable, and that more work is needed to promote high standards and to enhance the powers and the information resources available to clinical governance teams in hospital trusts and PCTs. The National Audit Office (NAO) reached similar conclusions in its 2003 report on clinical governance in secondary care[48] and in a recently published report on primary care[49], as did the review of clinical governance in Chapter 2 of *Good doctors, safer patients*. All these documents confirm the point that good progress has been made in setting up the underlying **structures and processes** of clinical governance but that a more sustained effort is needed to embed the **cultural change** needed.

4.5 To sum up, the NHS has laid the essential foundations of clinical governance even if it has not yet achieved its full potential to transform the culture of the NHS and to instil a commitment to continuous quality improvement throughout every healthcare organisation. The Government therefore believes that the way forward lies in building on what has already been achieved, rather than starting again in a different place.

4.6 This chapter reviews recent developments in the implementation of clinical governance in the NHS and then considers the specific recommendations of the Shipman Inquiry and of the three inquiries relating to the detection and handling of poor performance. The final sections of the chapter consider particular issues for primary care and secondary care respectively.

Recent developments in clinical governance

4.7 The Department of Health has recently undertaken a review of the arrangements for providing clinical governance support to NHS organisations. The conclusions will be announced shortly, but the fieldwork undertaken by the review confirmed that NHS organisations still perceive a need for dedicated support, both for training in clinical governance principles and processes and for help with specific local problems. The Department will be looking to make the best use of existing organisations to meet this need both nationally and locally.

4.8 In primary care, the Department, in collaboration with NHS Primary Care Contracting, issued in May 2006 a clinical governance framework to help PCTs develop detailed local criteria to assess the standard and quality of primary care dental services[50]. More generally, PCTs will wish to make use of the diagnostic information and guidance which the NAO has recently issued, based on the fieldwork for the study described at para 4.4 above.

4.9 One key component of clinical governance is the participation of health professionals in clinical audit. Following a recommendation in *Good doctors, safer patients* a clinical audit advisory group will be set up to help drive the further development of local and national clinical audit. This can potentially provide information both to benchmark the performance of healthcare organisations and to support the revalidation of individual clinicians, as discussed further in *Trust, assurance and safety* at para 2.25.

Identifying potential issues: the use of information sources

Kerr/Haslam Inquiry p30: Themes and trends arising from the data of complaints, incidents, patient and carer feedback should be analysed on a regular basis. This should form part of clinical governance and used to give early warning of emerging patterns of risk behaviour, in the interests of patient safety.

Ayling Inquiry para 2.45: The regular reports on patient complaints and concerns made to NHS Trust Boards and other corporate governance bodies should be structured to provide an analysis not only of trends in subject matter and clinical area but also to indicate whether a named practitioner has been the subject of previous complaints.

Neale Inquiry recommendation 22: Complaints handling should be aligned to quality management and patient services rather than claims management.

4.10 If healthcare provider organisations and PCTs are to fulfil their responsibilities for promoting the quality of the services they provide or commission, it is essential that they should identify and address any possible problems with professional behaviour or competence at the earliest possible stage. To do so, they need to scrutinise a range of routine indicators and to combine this with "opportunistic" information from sources such as complaints, concerns from fellow professionals – including those from other disciplines and sectors – and clinical negligence litigation. Other local organisations, such as other healthcare providers and the Healthcare Commission, may have complementary information. Healthcare organisations[viii] need to ensure that they have both the capacity to carry out these functions and the analytical tools to bring the information together.

4.11 For the medical profession, *Good doctors, safer patients* introduced the concept of the "GMC affiliate", a respected doctor who would work alongside lay associates and local clinical governance leads to investigate potentially serious issues of professional performance[51]. The Government has now decided to pilot this concept by introducing GMC affiliates in each strategic health authority, or in some cases also at sub-regional level (see *Trust, assurance and safety*, Chapter 3). The GMC affiliate will have a key role in ensuring that information from various sources and held in different healthcare organisations is, where necessary, brought together to give a fuller view of potential problems[ix]. Where the GMC affiliate concludes that there is a performance issue but that it is not sufficiently serious to require referral to the GMC centrally, one option would be to issue a "recorded concern" which would be entered on the medical register and brought to the attention of relevant employers and PCTs.

4.12 Later chapters in this response discuss specific sources of information – complaints and concerns (Chapter 5) and routine quality indicators (Chapter 8) – and *Trust, assurance and safety* discusses the complementary use of appraisal and revalidation. This chapter considers the

---

viii For convenience the term "healthcare organisations" will be used in this chapter to refer to PCTs in relation to the primary care contractors with whom they contract and to secondary care trusts in relation to the professional staff which they employ.

ix This would have been particularly helpful in the case of Clifford Ayling, where the failure to share information between the hospital employing Dr Ayling and the primary care organisation responsible for his GP contract resulted in lengthy delays in identifying the need for action.

processes which healthcare organisations need to follow to investigate potential concerns, whatever the original source; and to take effective action both to protect patients and (wherever possible) to help health professionals to remedy weaknesses. The general principles will be familiar to NHS organisations, but as part of the action programme needed to follow through the recommendations of the inquiries **the Department will consider with NHS and other stakeholders what further guidance would be helpful**.

Shipman Inquiry recommendation 4: There should be statutory recognition of the importance of the proper investigation of complaints to the processes of clinical governance and of monitoring the quality of health care.

4.13 The Department of Health fully agrees the need for healthcare organisations to make full use of information from complaints, alongside other potential sources of information, both in identifying professionals whose competence or behaviour may be a source of concern and for clinical governance purposes more widely. The positive use of complaints and feedback as a learning tool is already a well-established clinical governance process, and we are encouraging the sharing of insights within health communities so that other providers can share in the learning.

4.14 All NHS organisations are subject to a statutory "duty of quality"[52] which they discharge by complying with national standards as set out in *Standards for better health*, including ensuring that they have effective clinical governance processes in place. In secondary care the NHS Redress Act 2006 can require trusts, among other things, to report back to patients on the action which is being taken to prevent similar cases arising; and to prepare and publish an annual report about cases covered by the Act and lessons to be learnt from them[53]. However, given the emphasis that the Shipman Inquiry placed on the effective handling of complaints, and the similar recommendation in *Good doctors, safer patients*, **the Government will consider how this statutory responsibility could be further strengthened and extended to independent and third sector healthcare providers**. For instance,

- a requirement could be placed on each chief executive of a healthcare organisation (including commissioning organisations and provider organisations in the independent and voluntary sectors) to produce and publish an annual report to its board on the lessons learned from medical errors and complaints and the action that has been put in place as a result;

- in the NHS, all new chief executives currently receive a letter underlining their personal responsibilities in relation to the organisation's finances; this could be extended to spell out an equivalent personal responsibility for ensuring quality and safety.

We will develop detailed proposals in consultation with stakeholders as part of the wider package of legislation needed to implement the key proposals of *Trust, assurance and safety*.

Investigation of complaints and concerns and subsequent handling

Investigation of complaints and concerns

Shipman Inquiry recommendation 9: All 'clinical governance complaints' (save those which do not involve serious issues of patient safety and where the underlying facts giving rise to the complaint are clear and undisputed) should be referred to the inter-PCT investigation team. The objective of the investigation should be to reach a conclusion as to what happened and to set out the evidence and conclusions in a report which should go to the PCT with responsibility for the doctor. If the investigators are unable to reach a conclusion about what happened because there is an unresolved conflict of evidence, they should say so in their report.

Ayling Inquiry para 2.72: We recommend that SHAs work together with the Department of Health to produce guidance for PCTs and other NHS Trusts in handling such incidents [ie incidents involving potentially criminal activity], particularly since the latest reorganisation of the NHS has created a large number of relatively inexperienced PCTs with responsibility for GP contracts.

Kerr/Haslam Inquiry p27: Dedicated staff should be properly trained to carry out the investigations [of allegations of sexualised behaviour]. This relates closely to the recommendations we make at the end of Chapter 33 regarding investigations generally.

Kerr/Haslam Inquiry p31: Those who are given the task of responding and initiating any investigation should themselves be adequately trained, equipped with the necessary skills to carry matters forward, and of such seniority as to ensure that barriers and resistance are overcome.

Kerr/Haslam Inquiry p31: Current regulations should be amended to ensure that it is the duty of complaints officers to investigate complaints in a speedy, efficient and effective manner.

Kerr/Haslam Inquiry p32: Guidance issued under the regulations should clarify what constitutes a full and rigorous investigation, most notably that complaints officers be placed under a duty to raise additional issues for investigation.

4.15 The Department fully accepts the need for concerns relating to potential performance issues, whether they arise from internal clinical governance systems or from external complaints and expressions of concern, to be investigated and addressed professionally and objectively. As a matter of good practice, healthcare organisations should ensure that they have access for this purpose to trained investigators employed by or contracted to the organisation[x]. In relation specifically to complaints, the existing health standards already require all healthcare providers to operate systems that respond appropriately to complaints, and the Department will shortly be consulting on how these standards could be further strengthened (see next chapter, para 5.10).

x For patient safety investigations, healthcare organisations will also have access to the specialist safety investigator in the SHA's patient safety action team – see para 2.16 above.

Acting on the results of investigations

Shipman Inquiry recommendation 10: On receipt of the [investigation] report, the PCT group which carried out the second triage should consider what action to take. It might be appropriate to refer the matter to another body, such as the GMC or the NCAS. Alternatively, it might be appropriate for the PCT to take action itself, eg by invoking its list management powers. If the report of the investigation team is inconclusive, because of a conflict of evidence, the case should be referred to the Commission for Healthcare Audit and Inspection (now known as the Healthcare Commission), under a power which should be included in the amended draft Complaint Regulations when implemented.

4.16 We agree that it is vital for healthcare organisations to establish fair and transparent processes which balance the need to protect patients and the rights of health professionals to fair treatment, and which maintain a clear separation between investigation and subsequent decisions on handling. As already noted, the Department issued guidance relating to disciplinary procedures for employed doctors and dentists in 2005, and a possible model for general practice care has been developed by NCAS[54]; as already noted, NCAS is already available to give advice to employers and PCTs in individual cases and to carry out clinical assessments as required. **We will issue further guidance on the processes to be adopted in primary care as part of the guidance referred to in para 4.12 above**.

Kerr/Haslam Inquiry p34: Early consideration should be given to extending the remit of the NCAS to cover other healthcare professionals, particularly those providing care and treatment in mental health services.

4.17 A multi-agency working group set up under the auspices of the Chief Nursing Officer and in collaboration with NCAS has published a set of principles for handling concerns about professional performance[55]. This document is intended for use in all healthcare settings and for all health professions, and will help achieve consistency and fairness for staff while ensuring patient safety. **The Department and NCAS are now considering**, in the light of this publication and the recent patient safety report (see para 2.16 above), **the possible extension of the remit of NCAS to other professions**.

Possible escalation to the Healthcare Commission or other bodies

Shipman Inquiry recommendation 13: The draft Complaints Regulations, when implemented, should include a power enabling PCTs to refer a complaint to the Health Commission for investigation at any point during the first stage of the complaints procedures. Cases raising difficult or complex issues or involving issues relating to both primary and secondary care might be referred to the Healthcare Commission for investigation at the time of the second triage, or later if the investigation by the inter-PCT investigation team raises more complex issues than had initially been apparent. Referral to the Healthcare Commission should also take place in cases where the inter-PCT investigation team has found that it cannot reach a conclusion because there remain unresolved disputes of fact. The purpose of the referral would be for the Healthcare Commission to carry out any further necessary investigation, and, if appropriate, to set up a panel to hear oral evidence about the facts in dispute and to decide where the truth lay.

Kerr/Haslam Inquiry p32: Chief Executives acting on the advice of their complaints managers should be given the authority to refer a complaint to the Healthcare Commission for further consideration.

4.18 We agree in principle that there could be advantage in providing some resource to help healthcare organisations with the most complex investigations, especially those involving patient safety incidents (see para 2.16) or health professionals working across more than one organisation. A number of health communities have already developed specialist investigative capacity of this kind (see para 4.34 below).

4.19 The Government is not convinced that it would be appropriate to give an automatic right for frontline healthcare organisations to refer complex complaints to the Healthcare Commission; this would undermine the drive to improve the skills and capacity of healthcare organisations to meet their own requirements, and would distract the Healthcare Commission from its primary responsibility to ensure and assess the safety and quality of organisations as a whole. However, there may be occasions in which the investigation of performance issues relating apparently to a single individual may indicate some deeper structural problems in the organisation. In these circumstances, it would be entirely appropriate for NHS bodies to alert the Healthcare Commission, and in turn for the Commission to investigate those incidents which meet its investigation criteria.

Overlapping investigations

Shipman Inquiry recommendation 7 (contd): [Clinical governance] complaints should be referred for a further triage (the second triage) to a small group comprising two or three people – for example, the Medical Director or Clinical Governance Lead, a senior non-medical officer of the PCT and a lay member of the PCT board. The object of the second triage should be to decide whether the complaint is to be investigated by or on behalf of the PCT or whether it should instead be referred to some other body, such as the police, the GMC or the NCAS.

Recommendation 11: Neither an intention on the part of the complainant to take legal proceedings, nor the fact that such proceedings have begun, should be a bar to the investigation by a NHS body of a complaint. In circumstances where the NHS body is taking disciplinary proceedings relating to the subject matter of the complaint against the person complained of, a complainant should be entitled to see the report of the investigation on which the disciplinary proceedings are to be based and should not merely be informed that the investigation of his/her complaint is to be deferred or discontinued.

Recommendation 12: In some circumstances, it may be necessary for a NHS body to defer or discontinue its own investigation of a complaint if the matter is being investigated by the police, a regulatory body, a statutory inquiry or some other process. However, a NHS body should never lose sight of its duty to find out what has happened and to take whatever action is necessary for the protection of the patients of the doctor concerned. It should also provide such information to the complainant as is consistent with the need, if any, for confidentiality in the public interest. The relevant provisions of the draft Complaints Regulations should be amended to reflect these principles.

Ayling Inquiry para 2.71: There should be set out in a Memorandum of Understanding (such as exists between the GMC and the NCAS) between the NHS, professional regulatory bodies such as the GMC and the CPS a clear agreement as to the responsibilities of each organisation in the investigation of potential criminal activity by health care professionals. This should then be promulgated to the NHS and built into the guidance suggested below.

Kerr/Haslam Inquiry p32: Current regulations should be amended, and suitable guidance prepared, to allow and ensure that complaints managers consider the reference of any complaint received which, if true, would disclose the commission of a crime, to the local police force.

Kerr/Haslam Inquiry p32: Complainants should be allowed to pursue litigation at the same time as a complaint is being investigated.

4.20 Current procedures may lead to a series of investigations by a range of different bodies – for example, the initial complaints manager in the primary care practice, the PCT or employer, and regulatory bodies. From the perspective of both the patient and the subject of the complaint this can lead to unnecessary lengthening of the time required to deal with it. It can also result in wasteful duplication and delays.

4.21 We believe that, as far as is practicable in individual cases, there should be a single investigation. The manager initially assigned to investigate should be required to identify from the outset the other organisations that might have an interest, to alert them to the issues, and (with support from the PCT or – for doctors – the GMC affiliate, as appropriate) to agree handling.

4.22 If the results of a local investigation are to be usable by other bodies, eg the professional regulatory organisations, it is vital that they are carried out to acceptable standards, for instance in relation to evidence gathering. For this reason, as announced in para 4.17 of *Trust, assurance and safety*, **the Government will be inviting CHRE to advise on protocols for local investigations and on the criteria for referring issues on to the regulatory bodies**.

4.23 We agree that, even where the police, the NHS counter-fraud service or a regulatory body have taken over the lead responsibility for investigating the issues arising out of a complaint, the PCT or employer retains responsibility for protecting patients locally and for keeping the complainant informed as far as possible. Advice relating to investigations involving the police, the Health and Safety Executive and the NHS has recently been issued in the form of a Memorandum of Understanding (MOU)[56] and the GMC and Nursing and Midwifery Council have agreed a similar MOU with the police and the Crown Prosecution Service.[57]

4.24 We agree that legal proceedings, or the threat of legal proceedings, should not prevent a PCT or employer from continuing to investigate a complaint, provided that they can do so without prejudicing the legal proceedings. We also agree that the complainant should have access to the factual findings of any investigation, whether or not possible litigation is being considered. **We will give further guidance on all these issues, after consultation with stakeholders, as part of the guidance referred to at para 4.12 above**.

> Ayling Inquiry para 2.73: We further recommend that part of the guidance we have suggested SHAs and the Department of Health develop for the NHS [for investigating incidents involving potentially criminal activity] should specifically address a patients communications strategy and the involvement of local victim support services.

4.25 The Government fully agrees that it is vital, during and after the investigation of any serious allegations or concerns, to communicate information about the progress of the investigation as fully as possible to the patients concerned, their families, and where appropriate the general public. The Government also agrees that local victim support services may play a key role. We will ensure that all these points are covered in the guidance referred to above.

Specific issues in primary care

4.26 Primary care services in the NHS are, and have been since the beginning of the NHS, highly devolved: most primary medical care is provided by a large number of independent contractors, the great majority of whom work in small practices with typically only 5-10 clinical staff under contract to a PCT. Arrangements for the other primary care contractors (dentists, pharmacists, optometrists) are broadly similar, although an increasing proportion of pharmacists and optometrists now work for large chains with their own internal clinical governance arrangements.

4.27 Even today, the main contact that most people have with health services is with their local GP, dentist or pharmacist. As more care is shifted into community settings and primary care practices begin to take a larger role in commissioning services (see para 2.20 above), the role of primary care will become even more important. Confidence in primary care practitioners is therefore central to sustaining public and patient confidence in health professionals as a whole.

4.28 This section focuses in particular on general medical practitioners, although similar principles apply to the other primary care professions. The vast majority of GPs fulfil their responsibilities with dedication and professionalism, leading by example and going the extra mile to ensure high standards of patient care. But for a very small minority – doctors who may be suffering from health problems, under pressure, or in danger of losing touch with their core professional values – the high levels of autonomy and influence which their position brings can result in especial risk for patients. One of the themes running through the Shipman Inquiry is the extent to which colleagues, patients

– even the local police force – were unable to entertain the possibility that a respected GP could be capable of deliberate harm to his patients, even when the warning signals were so clear. Local clinical governance systems therefore have to be resilient enough to identify such cases, rare as they are, and ensure that effective action is taken.

4.29 All primary care practices are required, as noted above, to have a clinical governance lead and clinical governance systems. But it is not always easy for practice partners to appreciate that a colleague's performance is becoming unsafe, and even if they see the warning signs they may be reluctant to take action. And a minority of GPs, some 6.6% in England in September 2005, still practise as single-handers. PCTs therefore have a key role, as explained in Chapter 2, both for promoting and supporting clinical governance in individual contractors and for providing the ultimate "safety net" of assurance that contractors are safe and fit for purpose.

4.30 Recent developments in the NHS, as summarised in *Creating a patient-led NHS* and *Commissioning a patient-led NHS*, have impacted on PCTs in three main ways:

- the number of PCTs have been reduced by about 50% since the Shipman Inquiry report was written (from 303 to 152), and they cover much larger populations (typically populations of 500,000 or more rather than the previous 100,000 to 200,000). This could result in PCT officers becoming more "distant" from practices and having less direct local knowledge. It will however have the major advantage of enabling PCTs to build up specialist expertise in handling performance issues;

- there is a continuing development programme to strengthen PCTs' structures, systems, processes and capacity for commissioning services. There could be useful synergies between the skills and processes needed to commission for quality in secondary care and the management of primary care contracts;

- more services will be provided in primary and community care settings and there will be an increasing variety of types of provider organisation, including new types of private and voluntary sector providers. These will include nurse-led community services, specialist out-of-hours providers, and community health centres and community hospitals offering a mix of primary and secondary health services. PCTs will need to ensure comparable standards across these different kinds of provider. This may require new approaches to performance management, including the use of new PCT contractual freedoms such as those announced in *Our health, our care, our say*[58] to drive up quality and responsiveness through contestability. **The Department will provide support and guidance as needed, for example recent guidance on clinical governance safeguards for practice-based commissioning[59] and guidelines to be published shortly on accrediting GPs and pharmacists with special interests.**

These and other significant developments both increase the scale of the challenge facing PCTs and strengthen their capacity to meet that challenge.

Accountability of GPs to PCTs

4.31 *Good doctors, safer patients recommended that*

> Further attention should be paid to ensuring the formal and personal accountability of individual general practitioners to their primary care trust, through use of standard contracts and other mechanisms. In particular, primary care trusts should be guaranteed unfettered access to all patient records.[60]

Formally, GPs are already accountable to PCTs – as members of a practice, through the practice contract; and as individuals, through the list management arrangements described in para **2.8** above. As announced in Chapter 2 of *Trust, assurance and safety* the Department of Health will be discussing with stakeholders how professional standards could be included in GP contracts[61].

4.32 However, this accountability is meaningless unless PCTs can effectively monitor the quality of services provided by primary care practices, including monitoring the patterns of complaints against individual GPs, and can investigate effectively when there is cause for concern. The Government therefore supports the principle that PCTs should have access to patient records where required in the context of an investigation. **We will ensure that this is an unambiguous contractual obligation for all GPs, if necessary by clarifying the regulations which specify the mandatory elements of General Medical Services and Personal Medical Services contracts.** As part of the work to develop common protocols for local investigations (see para 4.22) we will agree with stakeholders the criteria for such access and the safeguards under which it will be exercised, building on the existing code of practice[62].

4.33 Access to information on complaints is discussed in the next chapter and routine monitoring information in Chapter 8.

PCT capacity to investigate clinical governance issues

Shipman Inquiry recommendation 8: The investigation of 'clinical governance complaints' should not be undertaken by PCT staff. Instead, groups of PCTs should set up joint teams of investigators, who should be properly trained in the techniques of investigation and should adopt an objective and analytical approach, keeping their minds open to all possibilities.

4.34 Many PCTs have already experimented with common service agencies, serving groups of up to 10 PCTs, to provide a "critical mass" for handling performance issues and related remedial education. However, these arrangements can have problems of their own, as a recent report by the Sheffield School of Health and Related Research (ScHARR)[63] has demonstrated. And PCTs, as already noted, are now in general larger and may in some cases be able on their own to provide the expert capacity needed. The Department does not therefore intend to be prescriptive about the best way in which PCTs should secure the investigative capacity they need, although it will commend the "multi-PCT" model as one option. For patient safety incidents, as noted above, support will be available from the specialist investigator in the SHA's patient safety action team.

PCT powers to deal with poorly performing practices or individuals

Shipman Inquiry recommendation 19: The powers of PCTs should be extended so as to enable them to issue warnings to GPs and to impose financial penalties on GPs in respect of misconduct, deficient professional performance or deficient clinical practice which falls below the thresholds for referral to the GMC or exercise of the PCT's list management powers.

Recommendation 27: The Family Health Services Appeals Authority (Special Health Authority) or its proposed successor, the NHS Litigation Authority, should collect and analyse information relating to the use made by PCTs of their list management powers. Such analysis would assist the DoH in providing guidance to PCTs about the types of circumstance in which they might properly use their powers.

Recommendation 28: The Government should consider the feasibility of providing a financial incentive for the achievement of GP practice accreditation by means of a scheme similar to that operated by the Royal College of General Practitioners in Scotland.

4.35 PCTs will in future have a wider range of options for dealing with performance issues in health professionals or practices in contract with them, including

- the new arrangements for the regulation of the healthcare professions announced in *Trust, assurance and safety* – in particular, the development of the network of "GMC affiliates" and of the use of recorded concerns (see para 4.11), and the development of the GMC register as the key central repository for information on the registration status and any disciplinary issues relating to individual doctors (see para 8.7);

- the system of registration of healthcare providers by the new regulator for health and adult social care announced in *The future regulation of health and adult social care in England* (see para 2.5).

In the light of these changes, and as announced in Chapter 3 of *Trust, assurance and safety*[64], **the Department will during 2007 review the Performers List arrangements**.

4.36 The Department agrees that it would be helpful for PCTs to have a range of sanctions available to them to deal with performance that falls short of requiring use of the list management powers. We are particularly attracted to two of the ideas put forward in the Shipman Inquiry's seminars:

- constructive measures such as a requirement to undergo training and/or to give a written undertaking for specific improvements in performance

- a graded series of formal warnings

provided that these were backed up as necessary by the ultimate use of the list management powers or any future equivalent. **We will take forward these ideas in consultation with NHS, NCAS and professional organisations, as part of the review of the Performers List referred to above**. We are less convinced that the case for financial penalties has been made but will discuss this also with stakeholders.

4.37 The Family Health Services Appeal Authority (FHSAA) does already collect some statistics on PCTs' use of their powers; for instance, in its annual report for the year ending 31 March 2005, the FHSAA reported that it was notified of 73 suspensions, 66 removals and 12 contingent removals[65]. It also noted that

> "The largest growth in notifications relates to GPs. Interestingly, and despite the growth in notifications, the number of appeals has not grown proportionately which suggest decisions at local level are becoming more assured and less vulnerable to challenge."

4.38 The report by ScHARR already referred to analysed PCTs' handling of cases involving a criminal conviction or caution. ScHARR concluded that PCTs seemed in general to be well informed about the options open to them and that "although [such cases] were rare ... they can be and are handled within a set of tried, tested, well supported and performance-managed procedures". In the light of this evidence, the Department does not consider that it would be reasonable to impose additional reporting requirements on PCTs, although it will consider a follow-up to the ScHARR study once the new PCTs have settled in.

4.39 Voluntary systems of accreditation, such as that developed by the Royal College of General Practitioners, are a very effective way of encouraging already good practices to aspire to even higher standards. Even with financial incentives, however, there must be some doubt as to whether voluntary accreditation would have sufficient impact on the least motivated practices, where defective professional performance is most likely to be found. The Government therefore considers that all providers of healthcare (including in principle primary medical care practices) should be registered under the new arrangements for ensuring safety and quality (see para 2.5 above). We are currently consulting on ways in which this could be achieved and will announce further details in due course.

PCT support for practices

Shipman Inquiry recommendation 30: PCTs should be willing and able to provide advice to GP practices on good recruitment practice and should also be willing to offer support in drafting job specifications and advertisements. They should be prepared, if requested, to assist in sifting applications (if multiple applications are received) and in making the necessary checks on applications before the interview stage, so as to exclude in advance any applicants who are unsuitable. However, this latter exercise may be too much of a burden for PCTs unless and until the Inquiry's recommendations for greater information to be placed on the GMC's website and for the creation of a central database of information about doctors (see below) are implemented.

Recommendation 31: A standard reference form should be developed for use in connection with appointments to GP practices. PCTs should insist that a reference is obtained from the doctor's previous employer or PCT. In the case of a PCT, the reference should be signed by the Medical Director or Clinical Governance Lead.

Recommendation 32: When recruiting a new member, GP practices should canvass and take account of the views of their patients about the kind of doctor the practice needs.

4.40 The Department agrees in principle that PCTs should offer help to primary care practices in making appointments, including the checks referred to in Chapter 3 above, and will discuss with NHS, professional and patient organisations how they can best be implemented. Any support for practices should be given on request and should not be mandatory.

4.41 The Department agrees that practices should be responsive to the views of their patients in deciding how to develop their services. Ultimately however practices must remain accountable for the way in which those services are provided, including any new appointments.

Small and single-handed practices

Shipman Inquiry recommendation 29: The policy of the DoH and PCTs should be to focus on the resolution of the problems inherent in single-handed and small practices. More support and encouragement should be given to GPs running single-handed and small practices. In return, more should be expected of such GPs in terms of group activity and mutual supervision. Initiatives such as the sharing of staff, mentoring and peer support schemes that promote the 'cross-fertilisation' of staff between one single-handed or small GP practice and another should be encouraged wherever possible. The DoH should take responsibility for these initiatives.

Ayling Inquiry para 2.48: We therefore recommend that PCTs should develop specific support programmes for single-handed practitioners, to be agreed with the practitioner concerned and the PCT's Strategic Health Authority. Such programmes should pay critical attention to managing the risks of clinical and professional isolation associated with single-handed practice. Implementation should be monitored by the Strategic Health Authority and form part of the regular CHAI [Healthcare Commission] review of the PCT.

Ayling Inquiry para 2.49: Additionally, PCTs should pay particular attention to developing and supporting the independence of practice managers in single-handed practices, including the acknowledgment and resolution of potential conflicts of interest which may arise where the manager is the spouse or a close relative of the practitioner. This too should be the subject of monitoring and review by Strategic Health Authorities and [the Healthcare Commission].

4.42 As the inquiry itself recognised, many small or single-handed practices deliver excellent services. Nevertheless, the Department accepts that practitioners working single-handed or in small practices are at particular risk of becoming professionally isolated. The Department is therefore sympathetic to the intention behind these recommendations **and will discuss further with NHS and professional organisations how they could be carried forward**.

Specific issues in secondary care

Kerr/Haslam Inquiry p23: Procedures and policies should be put in place, within twelve months of the publication of this Report, to ensure that all NHS organisations are aware of the therapies being undertaken by all staff, particularly those where patients believe clinical governance committees should be aware of them and making decisions about their use.

p24: Within mental health services no member of the health care team should be permitted to use or pursue new or unorthodox treatments without discussion and approval by the team (such approval to be recorded in writing).

p24: The full range of physical, psychological and complementary therapies used by mental health professionals should be recorded and discussed through appraisal/job plans. Trusts should have a clear evidence base and protocols for guiding the use of these treatments.

4.43 In the Government's view, clinical governance committees should be aware of all "new and unorthodox treatments" in use within the healthcare organisation, whether in mental health or in other sectors. For instance, clinicians wishing to use novel surgical or other invasive treatments are required to take account of guidance from NICE's interventional treatments programme on the evidence of the safety and effectiveness of the proposed treatment. NICE is currently consulting on a new Methods Guide for the interventional procedures programmel[66]. This includes guidance to clinicians on the principles to follow when carrying out a new procedure, including informing their clinical governance lead. The final guide will be published in summer 2007. **In parallel with this, the Department of Health will update guidance to clinical governance committees on the steps needed to ensure patient safety in adopting innovative treatments.**

Chapter 5
Complaints and Concerns

5.1 This chapter considers the recommendations of the four inquiries on the handling of complaints and concerns. The Department fully accepts, as emphasised in the previous chapter, the important role which complaints and concerns can play as an integral part of an effective structure of clinical governance. Complaints from patients and concerns from fellow professionals may be the first signals drawing attention to deficient care or abuse of patients. Complaints handlers must therefore strike a careful balance – seeking to resolve the complaint, as far as possible, to the satisfaction of the complainant, but also being alert to the possible wider implications for patient safety.

5.2 The Shipman Inquiry's terms of reference were limited to primary care. We accept that there may be particular issues over the handling of complaints in primary care, where complaints staff may be working in greater isolation than their colleagues in secondary care. Nevertheless we need to work towards a complaints system which is easy for patients to understand and to navigate and which is fully integrated across primary and secondary care (and indeed also across the boundary between health and social care). This chapter therefore considers, where appropriate, the implications for complaints handling in other care settings.

Complaints: general approach

The 2004 complaints regulations

5.3 In January 2004, the Department of Health undertook a consultation exercise on a new set of complaints regulations. These regulations sought to provide a framework for future NHS complaints and to consolidate all amendments to the complaints process since the new system was introduced in 1996 into a single piece of secondary legislation. In particular, the proposed regulations would have:

- replaced the independent panel system with a truly independent review system, operated by the Healthcare Commission;

- aligned the systems for primary and secondary care and the independent sector;

- enabled patients and their representatives to complain directly to the PCT;

- introduced duties to provide a senior person to oversee the complaints process and to ensure that appropriate action is taken;

- introduced a duty to cooperate between and across the difference NHS sectors and between health and social care sectors;

- replaced the independent panel system with an independent review system, operated by the Healthcare Commission;

- introduced a duty in cross-boundary complaints to identify a 'lead' complaints manager, responsible for overall handling of the case; and

- placed an obligation on NHS bodies to ensure that staff who handle complaints are appropriately trained.

5.4 Following consultation, the Department decided to await publication of the Shipman Inquiry's fifth report before proceeding with all these proposed amendments. However, some of the more urgent changes were included in revised regulations which came into force in July 2004[67]. Under these regulations, local resolution procedures remained unchanged but the Healthcare Commission took responsibility for the independent review system (the second stage of the complaints process). Other amendments, relating to secondary care, widened the scope of matters falling within the NHS complaints procedure and provided for a senior person to oversee the complaints process.

The 2006 complaints regulations

5.5 Further amendments to the health and social care complaints regulations were introduced in September 2006[68]. Their main effect was to impose a reciprocal duty to cooperate on NHS bodies and local authorities; this provides for the transfer to the appropriate local authority of complaints made to NHS bodies that relate wholly or in part to concerns over social care services. Other amendments

- allow NHS organisations to provide complaints handling services to one another and to designate people other than employees as complaints managers;

- increase the time limit for an NHS body to respond to a complaint from 20 to 25 days and provide for the complainant to agree a longer period. This allows for a more thorough investigation of complex complaints rather than insisting on a fixed time period for all complaints.

Further proposed changes

5.6 During 2006, following a commitment in the White Paper *Our health, our care, our say*, the Department launched a project to carry out a fundamental review of the complaints systems in both health and social care. The aim will be to complete the process begun with the 2004 and 2006 regulations and to develop by 2009 a comprehensive single complaints system across health and social care. The review has been carried out under the oversight of a policy forum with representation from the Healthcare Commission, the Commission for Social Care Inspection, the PALS, complaints staff, and the office of the health and local government Ombudsmen.

5.7 As part of this project, the Department commissioned a programme of research including a review of the literature and qualitative research with people using complaints services. Findings of this research include the following:

- there is a reluctance to make formal complaints – experiences have to be very bad before people are prepared to come forward with their views;

- the complaints system is not widely understood and perceived as lengthy and bureaucratic;

- some patients are particularly hesitant about making complaints about GPs directly to the practice, because they think that this could have serious consequences for their relation to their GP;

- positive feedback tends to be given informally rather than through formal channels.

5.8 The Department will shortly be issuing a consultation paper with proposals for a new complaints system. The intention is to create a system which delivers a stronger voice for patients, in line with the overall objectives of the Government's public sector reform programme, and which is

- demonstrably independent

- simple, integrated and consistent across organisations and agencies

- focused on the needs of patients and based on an understanding of the needs of patients, carers and staff

- staffed by well-trained people with sufficient seniority in their organisations to effect improvement

- supported by managers who are committed to learning from mistakes and to delivering specific and systematic changes to the organisations against which complaints are made.

5.9 The remainder of this chapter points to some of the proposed changes and their relation to relevant recommendations of the four inquiries.

Complaints: the inquiry recommendations

Standards for complaints handling

> Kerr-Haslam Inquiry p30: The NHS should, jointly with the appropriate National Standards body, produce a standardised complaints system to be implemented in all Trusts/organisations providing services to NHS patients.

5.10 The current NHS standards *Standards for better health* already require all NHS healthcare organisations to ensure that patients and their representatives "have clear access to procedures to register formal complaints ... and are assured that organisations act appropriately on any concerns". There are similar requirements in the National Minimum Standards[60] applying to organisations in the independent and voluntary sectors. As part of the consultation referred to above, **the Government will be seeking views on possible developments of the current health and social care standards relating to complaints handling, building on work already carried out with the Health Service Ombudsman and the Healthcare Commission**; and in particular on how the standards could underline the importance of achieving demonstrable improvements in services (outcome standards) and not just efficiency in handling (process standards).

5.11 Complete "standardisation" across all the different kinds of healthcare organisation may be neither practicable nor desirable. However, the Government accepts that complaints systems should as far as possible be broadly consistent between different parts of the health and social care system; this will be one of the major themes of the consultation paper referred to in para 5.8 above.

Initial handling of complaints

Neale Inquiry recommendation 23: The head of the unit dealing with complaints should be an appropriately trained manager.

Kerr-Haslam Inquiry p31: PALS and complaints staff should have direct access to a line manager at board level and to senior medical staff and should be appointed at middle management level.

5.12 The Department agrees that complaints handlers in PCTs or hospital trusts should be appointed at a sufficiently senior level and have appropriate training, and that they should have direct access to the member of the executive board with overall responsibility for clinical governance issues. The DH/NPSA guidance referred to in the previous chapter[55] emphasises that where a more junior member of staff is the first to receive the complaint or concern they should promptly inform someone of sufficient seniority within the organisation to take effective action.

5.13 We also agree that complaints handlers in PCTs and in specialist trusts have a vital need for training and support. Training courses are already available, and **we will work with stakeholders to determine what other steps may be needed**. We noted in the previous chapter the need for PCT frontline complaints handlers to have access to a properly trained investigative resource.

Shipman Inquiry recommendation 5: On receipt by a PCT of a complaint about a GP, a 'triage' (the first triage) of the complaint should be conducted by a member of the PCT's staff who is appropriately experienced and has access to relevant clinical advice. The object of the first triage should be to assess whether the complaint arises from a purely private grievance or raises clinical governance issues.

Recommendation 6: 'Private grievance complaints' should be dealt with by appropriately trained PCT staff. The objectives in dealing with such complaints should be the satisfaction of the patient and, where possible, restoration of the relationship of trust and confidence between doctor and patient.

Recommendation 7: 'Clinical governance complaints' should be investigated with the dual objectives of patient protection and satisfaction and fairness to doctors.

5.14 Triaging cases into those involving "private grievance" and "clinical governance" issues has some attractions, but as the inquiry itself recognised the boundary between the two is not always clear-cut. Apparent "private grievance" complaints may indicate more serious problems within the practice, or patients may be reluctant to put forward their real concern (eg an allegation of inappropriate sexualised behaviour) but may make a more trivial complaint in order to draw attention to their unease. Healthcare organisations should therefore regard all complaints as potentially serious. **We will discuss further with stakeholders how we could best promote good practice in NHS organisations in identifying the more serious complaints**.

5.15 Where a healthcare organisation is satisfied that a complaint does not raise any broader issues of patient safety, we agree that the objective should be wherever possible to restore the trust between patient and doctor.

Objective standards for judging complaints

> Shipman Inquiry recommendation 16: Objective standards, by reference to which complaints can be judged, should be established as a matter of urgency. These standards should be applied by those making the decision whether to uphold or reject a complaint and by PCTs and other NHS bodies when deciding what actions to take in respect of a doctor against whom a complaint has been upheld. When established, the standards by reference to which complaints are dealt with must fit together with the threshold by reference to which the GMC will accept and act upon allegations, so as to form a comprehensive framework.

5.16 As noted above (para 4.22) the Department is inviting CHRE to lead work on protocols for NHS investigations. **This will include guidance for NHS complaints handlers on the standards for judging complaints and the thresholds at which they should consider referral to the professional regulators.**

Complaints against private or voluntary sector organisations

> Shipman Inquiry recommendation 14: Complaints procedures in the private sector should be aligned as closely as possible with those in the NHS, so that a complainant who does not receive a satisfactory response to his/her complaint can proceed to a second stage of the complaints procedures to be conducted by the Healthcare Commission.

5.17 We agree that standards for complaints handling in the independent and voluntary sectors should be aligned with those in the NHS, and we will work with the representative organisations of the two sectors and with the Healthcare Commission to ensure this. Independent clinics and hospitals registered with the Healthcare Commission are already required to have a policy for dealing with complaints; and the complaints service established by the General Dental Council in 2006 also requires dental practices treating private patients to have arrangements for investigating and resolving patients' complaints. **The government will consider how the new framework for regulation of healthcare organisations, now subject to consultation (see para 2.5), can best be used to ensure that all healthcare providers have safe systems for complaints handling linked to broader clinical governance systems.** PCTs commissioning services from the independent and voluntary sectors on behalf of NHS patients can reinforce this through contracts.

Advising and supporting patients who are considering a complaint

> Shipman Inquiry recommendation 17. In order to ensure that, so far as possible, complaints about healthcare can reach the appropriate destinations, there should be a 'single portal' by which complaints or concerns can be directed or redirected to the appropriate quarter. This service should also provide information about the various advice services available to persons who are considering whether and/or how to complain or raise a concern. Advice must be provided for persons who are concerned about the legal implications of raising a concern.

5.18 We accept that many patients are confused about how and where to make a complaint on a healthcare matter, and in particular about the role of the regulatory bodies. This has many causes: the UK healthcare system itself is complex, and media coverage of high profile GMC cases may encourage patients to think that the regulatory bodies have a wider remit than is the case. In any case, most people see the NHS as a single system and assume – quite reasonably – that, once a complaint is lodged at any point, "the system" will deal with it.

5.19 The Department has already put in place independent support for people wishing to raise concerns or complaints. In particular, ICAS is available to advise anyone wishing to make a complaint using the NHS complaints procedure. It also provides specialist advocacy support to those least able to pursue a complaint themselves. ICAS advocates can explain the role of regulatory bodies and the NHS complaints process and help clients to focus on the key issues which they wish to raise. ICAS advocates can also refer clients to other local specialist support as needed, for instance bereavement support or specialist mental health advocacy, or to local voluntary sector agencies.

5.20 Not all patients however are aware of ICAS or will wish to use their services. We are therefore sympathetic to the Shipman Inquiry's proposal for a single "portal" for submitting complaints. Experience suggests that however well such a "portal" is advertised, patients will still continue to submit complaints by a variety of routes. **What is needed therefore is a set of common standards for all healthcare and regulatory bodies to ensure that, wherever a complaint is submitted, it is promptly redirected to the appropriate body.** Where possible agreement should be sought from the patient or the patient's representative, although there may be occasions on which an urgent referral is needed even without explicit consent in order to protect other patients (for instance, in cases of alleged abuse). In any case, the patient should be told where the complaint has been sent and why, and what support is available. **We will discuss the detailed options with stakeholders.**

Review of the new complaints system

Shipman Inquiry recommendation 18: About two years after the complaints regulations come into force in their entirety, an independent review should be commissioned into the operation of the new arrangements for advising and supporting patients who wish to make a complaint.

5.21 The Department agrees that it would be sensible to review all aspects of the new complaints procedures after a reasonable period of experience in their use, and **will in due course discuss with stakeholders, including patient and carer organisations, the best way in which this could be done.**

Complaints: specific issues in primary care

PCT involvement in complaints

Shipman Inquiry recommendation 1: I endorse the provision contained in the draft National Health Service (Complaints) Regulations, whereby patients and their representatives who wish to make a complaint against a general practitioner (GP) will be permitted to choose whether to lodge that complaint with the GP practice concerned or with the local PCT. I also endorse the provision extending the time limit for complaining from six to twelve months.

Recommendation 3: Draft regulation 30 of the draft Complaints Regulations, which would require GP practices to provide PCTs with limited information about complaints received by the practice at intervals to be specified by the PCT, should be amended. GP practice should be required to report all complaints to the PCT within, say, two working days of their receipt. The report should contain the original letter of complaint or, if the complaint was made orally, the practice's record of the complaint. The PCT should log the complaint for clinical governance purposes and, if it considers that the complaint raises clinical governance issues, it should 'call in' the complaint for investigation.

Kerr-Haslam Inquiry p31: The revised regulations should require that all formal complaints should be directed to designated complaints managers in PCTs and NHS Trusts. Formal complaints should be interpreted as any matter which the complainants would like to be treated as formal.

5.22 The Department of Health is committed to the principle that complaints are generally best resolved locally. Patients say[70] that when something goes wrong, they are looking for an apology and reassurance that action will be taken to ensure it will not happen to other people. This will be most effective when the apology is genuine and delivered by the organisation that gave rise to the complaint. Equally if an organisation is to learn from its mistakes and to take action to prevent them happening again, staff need if possible to hear the grievance at first hand. This is consistent with the approach which the Government has taken in the NHS Redress Act 2006.

5.23 Nevertheless we accept that there will be occasions when a patient is reluctant to complain locally for fear of jeopardising their future relationship with the healthcare team. This may be especially important in primary medical care, where the relationship between patient and doctor tends to be longer-term and more personal than in secondary care. We need to protect patients in this situation, while maintaining as far as possible the principle of local resolution. We therefore agree with the view of the Shipman Inquiry, and with the equivalent recommendation in *Good doctors, safer patients*, that in these circumstances there should be an alternative route open to complainants. Equally, the complaints handler in a practice may on occasion wish to seek support from the PCT if he or she suspects that the complaint may be a symptom of a wider problem, or if the patient appears to be behaving in an unreasonable way.

5.24 We also accept that some complaints may raise issues which go beyond the needs of the individual complainant and point to some more general issue of patient safety. Particularly within the relative isolation of primary care it is possible that the complaints manager may fail to spot the potential significance of such complaints, or may be reluctant to take action that could have serious implications for healthcare staff in the organisation. We agree that in these circumstances some additional oversight is needed to ensure patient safety, even if the original complainant is satisfied by the explanation offered locally.

5.25 The Department is therefore minded:

- **to amend further the complaints regulations to enable patients to make complaints directly to the local PCT**. Patients would however need to accept that they would not in general be able to maintain their anonymity – the principles of natural justice mean that health professionals should have the opportunity to respond to any specific allegations made against them;

- **to require practices to copy all complaints letters to the PCT within a set period. PCTs would be required to maintain an oversight of all the complaints received by practice and to be prepared to investigate any patterns or trends of concern**. Evidence presented to the inquiry showed that the volume of complaints is modest – there was an average of about one complaint per GP in 2003-04 – and we believe that this would be a reasonable additional precaution to ensure that "clusters" of complaints against individual practices or clinicians are not overlooked.

5.26 Where a complaint is made directly to the PCT, the complaints handling staff at the PCT will need to form a view on whether some broader patient safety issue is involved. Where it is, there should be a thorough investigation under the direction of the PCT in order to protect patients. If no general patient safety issue arises, PCT staff should seek – with the patient's agreement – to involve the practice's complaints handlers to the maximum extent in resolving the issues. The mere fact that the PCT is aware of the complaint and will be monitoring the outcome should give patients reassurance that the practice will not simply "whitewash" the issue or discriminate subsequently against them.

5.27 The Department will consult in due course on the proposed regulatory changes and associated guidance in relation to primary medical care; and on the possible application of these principles to other areas of primary care.

Implied complaints

5.28 Some patients choose not to make complaints against their practice, but simply to move to another practice. In these circumstances, the opportunity for learning could potentially be lost. *Good doctors, safer patients* therefore proposed that when a patient switches their registered GP without changing their address, the patient should be offered a confidential interview with a member of staff from the PCT at a place of their choosing. **The Government agrees with this recommendation and will develop further guidance for PCTs on how it could be put into effect**. Since PCTs have a duty to prepare and keep up to date practices' lists of NHS patients, it should be relatively straightforward for PCT staff to identify such cases.

Raising standards of complaints handling

Shipman Inquiry recommendation 2: Steps should be taken to improve the standard of complaints handling by GP practices.

5.29 The Department has published generic good practice guidance[71] which is applicable in primary care. In addition, as already noted (para 5.10) the Department of Health will shortly be seeking views on possible developments to the standards for NHS complaints handling, including in practices. Middlesex University already offers a training programme for NHS complaints staff.

5.30 We are also working to establish a national network of local complaints managers, across health and social care, to enable complaints staff to share best practice and to provide mutual support. Unlike in secondary care, complaints staff in primary care may be working in relative isolation from colleagues with whom to share thoughts and ideas. In these circumstances it may be particularly helpful to have the opportunity to discuss individual cases with another, perhaps more experienced, complaints manager. SHAs may also have a role in sharing good practice.

Concerns

Handling concerns from fellow professionals

> Shipman Inquiry recommendation 15: Concerns expressed about a GP by someone other than a patient or patient's representative (eg by a fellow healthcare professional) should be dealt with in the same way as patient complaints. Such concerns should be investigated (where necessary) by the inter-PCT investigation team or, in a case raising difficult or complex issues, by the Healthcare Commission. Consideration should be given to amending the relevant provisions of the draft Complaints Regulations to permit the Healthcare Commission to accept and investigate concerns referred to it by a PCT or healthcare body without the need for a reference from the Secretary of State for Health.

5.31 We agree that concerns expressed by fellow health professionals and other colleagues should be handled in a similar way to complaints from patients. Both the Shipman and Clifford Ayling cases demonstrate how harm to patients could have been averted at a much earlier point if concerns of this kind had been taken seriously.

Supporting those wishing to raise concerns

> Shipman Inquiry recommendation 34: Every GP practice should have a written policy, setting out the procedure to be followed by a member of the practice staff who wishes to raise concerns, in particular concerns about the clinical practice or conduct of a healthcare professional within the practice. Staff should be encouraged to bring forward any concerns they may have openly, routinely and without fear of criticism. In the event that a member of the staff of a GP practice feels unable to raise his/her concern within the practice, s/he should be able to approach a person designated by the PCT for the purpose. The contact details of that person should appear in the written policy. The designated person should make him/herself known to all practice staff working in the PCT area. PCTs should ensure, through training, that practice staff understand the importance of reporting concerns and know how to do so.
>
> Recommendation 35: The written policy should contain details of organisations from which staff can obtain free independent advice. If the 'single portal' is created, in whatever form, the policy should set out contact details of that also.
>
> Recommendation 36: It should be a statutory requirement for all private healthcare organisations to have a clear written policy for the raising of concerns. Steps should be taken to foster in the private sector the same culture of openness that is being encouraged in the NHS.

Recommendation 39: There should be some national provision (probably a telephone helpline) to enable any person, whether working within heath care or not, to obtain advice about the best way to raise a concern about a healthcare matter and about the legal implications of doing so. It might be possible to link this helpline with the 'single portal' previously referred to.

Ayling Inquiry para 2.63: Local Medical Committees (LMCs) should clarify their role in relation to supporting GPs to make it explicit that acting on the receipt of information about a GP which indicates patient safety is being compromised is not part of their role, and ensure that this is embedded in professional guidance from the GMC and medical defence organisations.

Para 2.64: We further recommend that if LMCs are the recipient of concerns about a practitioner's clinical conduct or performance, this information should be immediately passed on to the relevant PCT or professional regulatory body for appropriate investigation. This should be made known to their constituents. We believe that not doing this would leave professional members and staff of a LMC in the potential position of having failed to meet their own professional obligations.

Kerr/Haslam Inquiry p29: The Department of Health should review the effectiveness of whistleblowing policies and initiatives within NHS-funded organisations.

p29: As a matter of some urgency the NHS should clarify the context of the positive obligation of NHS staff to inform NHS management of concerns in relation to the suspicion of the abuse of patients.

p30: Frontline staff who receive complaints about issues which compromise patient safety – whether or not in the confines of a therapeutic disclosure – should be under an express obligation to report that matter to a complaints manager (in or beyond their own organisation) whether or not they work for the organisation named in the complaint.

p34: Those responsible for developing the curricula for education programmes of healthcare professionals should ensure that information about and discussion of the ethical responsibilities of healthcare professionals to bring poor performance to light is given due weight.

p36: All Strategic Health Authorities should set up a manned telephone Helpline (perhaps called a 'PatientLine'), where anonymised (or identified) concerns could be received and processed. Any information received through the Helpline should be logged and received in confidence (unless there is express identification of the caller), and if there is sufficient information disclosed, should be discussed with the relevant NHS Trust or PCT. Consideration should be given as to how this information could best be collated either regionally or nationally.

5.32 We fully agree with the need to support and protect all those wishing, in good faith, to raise concerns about the actions of a healthcare colleague. They should be invited in the first instance to share their concerns in confidence with local management and with their professional regulator, even though (as with patient complaints) it may subsequently be necessary for them to make specific allegations if their concerns are to be further investigated. They should also be kept fully informed of the decisions taken in consequence.

5.33 While these principles may be particularly important in primary care – where staff may be working with little other support closely alongside the colleague whose performance or behaviour is giving cause for concern – we consider that they should apply to staff working in all healthcare settings. **We therefore propose that *all* organisations providing services to the NHS should have a written policy setting out the procedures to be followed by staff wishing to raise concerns, and we will be discussing with stakeholders how this might best be achieved.**

5.34 Under current regulationsl[72] Local Medical Committees (LMCs) are responsible for considering any allegation made to them by one GP against another, and for reporting the outcome to the PCT if they conclude that there is cause for concern. In the Government's view it is important that the PCT should have an overview of all concerns raised about the conduct of performance of health professionals working under contract for them and should take the final decision on whether any further action is needed. In doing so, the PCT will of course wish to seek the views of the LMC (which may for instance be able to advise of any malicious allegations) and also of the GMC affiliate. **The Government will consult further with stakeholders and issue further guidance or amend the regulations as needed.**

5.35 We recognise that there are situations (not just in primary care) in which staff feel unable to raise their concerns with the organisation in which they work. In these circumstances, the PCT or SHA may have a role to play; **we will explore this in more detail with stakeholders.**

5.36 We agree that similar principles should apply in the independent and voluntary sectors and will consider how this could be best achieved in the new regulatory system which will apply to all healthcare providers (see para 2.5 above).

5.37 Current ethical guidance from the GMC and the other regulators make clear the duty of all health professionals to raise any concerns they have about the conduct, health or performance of a fellow professional, especially where this could put the safety of patients at risk. There is also helpful guidance from NCAS[73], which has been recently updated. **We will discuss with the professional regulatory bodies and universities how this duty can be further emphasised, especially in undergraduate education.**

> Shipman Inquiry recommendation 37: Consideration should be given to amending the Public Interest Disclosure Act 1998 in order to give greater protection to persons disclosing information, the disclosure of which is in the public interest.

5.38 Staff who disclose concerns to the Healthcare Commission are already protected by the Public Interest Disclosure Act, as the Commission is now a "prescribed person" as a result of the Health and Social Care (Community Health and Standards) Act 2003. **We will also be working with NHS organisations to draw up protocols under the Act which will provide further protection, eg for staff bringing concerns to the attention of the GMC.** Subject to further discussion with stakeholders, we are not convinced that it is necessary to amend the Public Interest Disclosure Act 1998 at this stage.

> Shipman Inquiry recommendation 38: Written policies setting out procedures for raising concerns in the healthcare sector should be capable of being used in relation to persons who do not share a common employment.

5.39 We recognise that there may be occasions when a health professional in one organisation needs to raise concerns in relation to a colleague in another, and agree that this should be reflected in the written policies referred to above.

Chapter 6
Boundary Transgressions

6.1 Both the Kerr/Haslam and Ayling inquiries concerned allegations of sexual assault on female patients over prolonged periods of time. There were significant differences in the circumstances:

- Kerr and Haslam were consultant psychiatrists and the assaults were on especially vulnerable patients suffering from mental illness who were likely to be particularly reluctant to come forward with complaints;

- in Ayling's case, the issue was over the apparently inappropriate use of intimate examinations.

But in each case there was a similar pattern of a reluctance on the part of the NHS authorities to take seriously the complaints and concerns that were raised or to entertain the possibility that a health professional could be abusing the trust of vulnerable patients in such a way. We appreciate the courage and persistence of those involved, in particular the victims of Kerr and Haslam, for bringing their experience into the public domain and for ensuring that effective action was, in the end, taken. Patients deserve better protection in the future.

6.2 Since then, the work of organisations such as Witness[74] has shown that sexual or other abuse of patients by health professionals is, regrettably, more frequent than previously supposed. Very broad-brush estimates in other countries suggest that the prevalence could be as high as 6-7% of health professionals[75]. In some cases, abuse can initially manifest or be disguised as a minor infringement of the proper "boundaries" of trust which should exist between professional and patient, and then progress imperceptibly to more serious abuse. For this reason, it is now common to treat abuse as an extreme form of "boundary transgression".

6.3 Determining policy and ethical principles in this area therefore needs to start with a careful definition of what should be the proper boundaries between professional and patient. In doing so, a difficult balance needs to be struck – allowing professionals to show patients empathy, respect, support and reassurance, but ensuring that this remains within the proper boundaries of the relation between professional and patient and does not risk an inappropriate and possibly damaging emotional attachment on either side.

Guidance on boundary transgressions and sexualised behaviour

Development of guidance

Ayling Inquiry para 2.30: The DH [should] convene an expert group under the auspices of the Chief Medical Officer to develop guidance and best practice for the NHS on this subject. The group should include the NHS Confederation, the RCOG, the RCGP (and other Colleges as appropriate, such as the Royal College of Psychiatrists), NCAS, CHRE, GMC and representatives of undergraduate and postgraduate medical education. The group should take advice from experience of dealing with sexualised behaviour elsewhere in the public sector such as educational services and from health care systems in other countries such as Canada.

Kerr/Haslam Inquiry p27: Tthe Secretary of State, within 12 months of the publication of this Report, should convene an expert group to develop guidance and best practice for the NHS on boundary setting, boundary transgression, sexualised behaviour, and all forms of abuse of patients, in the mental health services.

p28: The terms of reference of the expert group should not be restricted to sexualised behaviour between psychiatrists (or other mental healthcare professionals) and current patients, but should also address former patients.

p26: All Trusts should develop, within their Code of Behaviour, guidance to reduce the likelihood of sexualised behaviour, that is incorporated into the contracts of employment of those staff, or contracts of engagement for all other persons providing mental health services within the NHS.

p27: The NHS should convene an expert group to consider what boundaries need to be set between patients and mental health staff who have been in long-term therapeutic relationships, and how those boundaries are to be respected in terms of guidelines for the behaviour of health service professionals, and the provision of safeguards for patients.

p27: Detailed, and readily accessible, guidance should be developed for medical professionals. The guidance should be framed in terms which address conduct which will not be tolerated and which is likely to lead to disciplinary action. Such guidance, if not provided at a professional regulatory level, should be supplemented by the NHS at an employment level.

p27: Policies should be developed that enable health workers to feel able to disclose feelings of sexual attraction at the earliest stage possible without the automatic risk of disciplinary proceedings. Colleagues must also feel able to discuss openly and report concerns about the development of attraction/overly familiar relationships with patients. These policies should include all grade levels, including consultant.

6.4 The Government has invited CHRE to lead a project involving all relevant stakeholders – including voluntary organisations, healthcare and professional regulatory bodies, NHS and professional organisations – to develop a comprehensive suite of guidance in this area. The CHRE project will, among other things:

- produce detailed guidance for health professionals agreed by all the health professions regulators on boundary violations, including definitions of abuse and a discussion of risk behaviours in relation to their clinical context. This will build on and harmonise guidance already issued by individual regulators[76]. Guidance will set out agreed principles to define the proper boundaries which should be observed between professionals and patients and covering issues such as social and financial relationships, growing emotional attachment, and the period of time which must elapse after the end of a therapeutic relationship (if ever) before these precautions can be relaxed;

- develop guidance for members of the professional regulators' fitness to practice panels on the appropriate sanctions for different degrees of boundary violations;

- develop information for patients to raise their awareness of professional boundary issues, with particular attention to the special needs of vulnerable groups;

- building on the previous three publications, develop guidance for NHS and other healthcare employers on how to prevent, detect and investigate boundary violations, and how to respond effectively to patients' complaints in this area;

- develop educational standards on boundary issues for adoption into pre-registration training and continuous professional development for all health professionals; and

- review current research to determine the profile of perpetrators and possible predictors of abuse.

CHRE has been asked to complete this work by summer 2007.

Research on prevalence

> Kerr/Haslam Inquiry p28: There should be detailed research carried out and published by the Department of Health to show the prevalence of sexual assaults, sexual contact, or other sexualised behaviour, between doctors and existing and/or former patients – particularly in the field of mental health.
>
> p28: The Department of Health should urgently investigate and report upon the need for a co-ordinated method of mandatory data collection and mandatory recording, in relation to the area of abuse of patients by mental healthcare professionals.

6.5 As already noted, the CHRE project will review current research on the profile of people perpetrating boundary violations. **In the light of this review the Department of Health will consider whether to commission further comprehensive research on the prevalence of sexualised behaviour.** In the meanwhile, we will encourage the regulators to carry out a retrospective analysis of recent fitness to practise cases to determine in what proportion this has been a factor. All patient safety incidents, including abuse of patients by health professionals, should be reported to SHAs through the standing arrangements for serious untoward incidents. Once the CHRE project has completed its work **the Department of Health will consider whether the information received from these reports could be further categorised so as to allow routine analysis of this kind**.

Guidance to employers on handling allegations

Kerr/Haslam Inquiry p25: The Department of Health should develop and publish a specific policy, with practical guidance on implementation, to guide NHS managers in their handling of allegations or disclosure of sexualised behaviour. The policy should address the various issues and difficulties set out above and include examples of good practice, as well as the extended range of options for action that could be applied; where advice and assistance can readily be provided; guidance on record-making and keeping. The guidance should also include a range of preventative measures (for example, specific accessible information for patients on what they should and should not expect in consultations, and who they can speak to for confidential advice and assistance).

p32: Where possible, the NHS should give clear advice and guidance on employment protocols following allegations of abuse.

p34: Within 12 months of the publication of this Report the Department of Health should develop and publish national advice and guidance to Primary and Secondary Health Care Trusts addressing the [action to be taken by staff on the] disclosure of sexual, or other, abuse by patients or other service users, with particular emphasis on users of mental health services.

6.6 The Government accepts these recommendations and is asking CHRE to progress them as part of the project referred to in para 6.4 above.

Advocacy services

Ayling Inquiry para 2.34: We therefore recommend that accredited training should be provided for all PALS officers in this potential aspect of their work [complaints relating to sexualised behaviour], and that SHAs should require confirmation from each NHS Trust in their area of the completion of such training within the next 12 months.

Kerr/Haslam Inquiry p26: In relation to disclosures of alleged abuse, voluntary advocacy and advice services (independent of the NHS) should be supported by central public funding to offer advice and assistance to patients and former patients (particularly those who are mentally unwell, or who are otherwise vulnerable).

6.7 The Government agrees the importance of training for PALS officers in dealing with issues of alleged sexualised behaviour. The National PALS Development Group has developed a template to help SHAs establish local training needs.

6.8 Patients or their representatives who wish to raise complaints already have access to support from ICAS staff (see para **5.19** above). As a general principle, the Government believes that it is better to strengthen the competency of staff working in existing complaints advocacy services than to set up parallel arrangements for particular groups of patients.

6.9 The voluntary organisation Witness (see para 6.2 above) has already delivered training in issues relating to sexualised behaviour to mixed groups of some 60 ICAS and PALS staff, and this training has now been rolled out to many more staff nationwide. The service specification for the delivery of ICAS services now requires the provision of training in these issues.

Chaperoning policies

Ayling Inquiry para 2.58: We recommend that no family member or friend of a patient should be expected to undertake any formal chaperoning role. The presence of a chaperone during a clinical examination and treatment must be the clearly expressed choice of a patient. Chaperoning should not be undertaken by other than trained staff: the use of untrained administrative staff as chaperones in a GP surgery, for example, is not acceptable. However the patient must have the right to decline any chaperone offered if they so wish.

Para 2.59: Beyond these immediate and practical points, there is a need for each NHS Trust to determine its chaperoning policy, make this explicit to patients and resource it accordingly. This must include accredited training for the role and an identified managerial lead with responsibility for the implementation of the policy. We recognise that for primary care, developing and resourcing a chaperoning policy will have to take into account issues such as one-to-one consultations in the patient's home and the capacity of individual practices to meet the requirements of the agreed policy.

6.10 Comprehensive guidance on chaperoning for PCTs and primary care health professionals, covering these and other points, was issued by the Clinical Governance Support Team in June 2005[77]. The basic principles are applicable to health professionals working in all settings, **but the Government will discuss with the health professions regulators and with NHS Employers whether specific guidance on chaperoning in secondary care settings would be helpful**.

Ayling Inquiry para 2.60: Reported breaches of the chaperoning policy should be formally investigated through each Trust's risk management and clinical governance arrangements and treated, if determined as deliberate, as a disciplinary matter.

6.11 The Government agrees and will ask CHRE to draw this recommendation to the attention of all healthcare organisations as part of the suite of guidance described at para 6.4 above.

Chapter 7
Particular Issues In Mental Health Services

7.1 The problem discussed in the previous chapter – finding the right balance between giving patients reassurance and support while respecting the proper boundaries between professional and patient – is especially acute in mental health services.

7.2 Patients with mental illness are particularly vulnerable. Compared with other patients, they may be the least likely to be able to enter into an informed discussion with health professionals on treatment options and the most uncritical of the treatments proposed. Many patients with mental illness, particularly with chronic conditions, are at risk of becoming excessively dependent on their therapist and of forming an emotional attachment (which they may believe is reciprocated). Given all this, health professionals treating mental illness need to take particular care to maintain professional boundaries and to avoid any behaviours which could be misinterpreted or which could inadvertently harm their patients.

7.3 Where issues arise, patients with mental illness may also have particular difficulty in raising concerns – and when they do pluck up courage, they may well not be taken seriously. In the Kerr/Haslam case, it took the courage and persistence of a small number of victims over many years before the authorities took effective action. Once the issues came out in the open, a number of additional victims were encouraged to come forward who had previously kept silent either out of fear or out of a reluctance to re-open old wounds. PCTs and employers therefore need to show particular sensitivity in investigating allegations in this field.

7.4 This chapter looks at the recommendations of the Kerr/Haslam inquiry relating to the specific issues of mental health services.

Patient confidentiality

Kerr/Haslam Inquiry p26: Trusts' confidentiality policies should include a section on disclosure within therapeutic interactions in psychiatric practice and should be supported by inter-agency information-sharing policies to be used in all cases of patient abuse.

p27: The Secretary of State, within 12 months of the publication of this Report, should commission and publish guidance and issue advice and instruction (preferably in consultation with the professional regulatory bodies and healthcare Colleges) as to the meaning and limitations of patient confidentiality in mental health settings. Such guidance should be kept under regular review.

7.5 Guidance on the protection of vulnerable adults in health and social care settings makes clear the responsibility of all health and social care workers to report allegations of abuse, even if the information is disclosed in a therapeutic setting.[78] Health and social care organisations in turn are required to join in multi-agency arrangements and to take appropriate action to protect patients and the public[78], including where appropriate referring care workers who have been responsible for abuse to be included in the Protection of Vulnerable Adults (POVA) list[79].

7.6 The Government however recognises that some health professionals may be still be uncertain about the implications of patient confidentiality in relation to such allegations. **The Government therefore accepts in principle that further guidance on information sharing in mental health services would be helpful and is already working with the Royal College of Psychiatrists, the Information Commissioners and voluntary organisations to develop such guidance.** We expect to be able to publish the guidance in the spring.

Advocacy and advice

> Kerr/Haslam Inquiry p30: Health and social care commission[er]s should resource independent mental health advocacy as a priority.
>
> p31: The Department of Health should introduce permanent arrangements for the provision of independent advice for mental health patients.

7.7 Para 5.19 above has already referred to the important role which ICAS plays in advising patients who wish to raise a complaint or a concern; ICAS is specifically tasked with providing specialist advocacy support for patients least able to pursue a complaint for themselves; and the majority of ICAS advocates have now received training in the special needs of patients suffering from mental illness. In the Department's view, it would be better to reinforce the skills of ICAS advocates in helping patients with a variety of needs, rather than to superimpose a different set of arrangements just for patients with mental illness.

Supervision of consultant psychiatrists

> Kerr/Haslam Inquiry p33: The Department of Health in association with NIHME [the National Institute for Mental Health in England] and the Royal College of Psychiatrists should publish guidance in relation to clinical supervision of consultant and career grade psychiatrists.

7.8 The Government does not accept that the risks associated with autonomous clinical practice are different in kind in psychiatry from those in other clinical disciplines, or that consultant psychiatrists should be subject to clinical supervision. The general safeguards described in this document and in *Trust, assurance and safety* – in particular, strengthened clinical governance, a robust system of revalidation, and closer links between local clinical management and national regulators via the proposed GMC affiliates – should be sufficient to ensure that any poor practice or deliberate abuse is rapidly identified and dealt with, in psychiatry as in other disciplines.

Intervention by regulators

> Kerr/Haslam Inquiry p33: Any deviation from acceptable practice [in applying the principles of the new disciplinary framework for doctors] in mental health services should be identified by the relevant statutory regulatory body and, where appropriate, by Monitor, and a standard, fair and transparent set of rules governing conduct of all mental health NHS staff in all NHS bodies and Foundation Trusts be quickly established.

7.9 Trust boards, in mental health services as in other specialist trusts, have the primary responsibility of ensuring that good practice in relation to the new disciplinary framework for doctors is applied throughout the trust. Where the Healthcare Commission identifies any significant deviations in the course of its annual assessment of a trust, or in the course of an ad hoc investigation, we would expect it to draw this to the attention of the trust board and to Monitor or the SHA as appropriate. A prolonged failure to establish satisfactory disciplinary systems might well call the trust's registration into question, under the new regulatory framework described in *The future regulation of health and adult social care in England* (see para 2.5 above).

Education and training

> Kerr/Haslam Inquiry p34: The GP curriculum should be reviewed to ensure that sufficient focus is given to the needs, treatment and care of patients experiencing mental health problems and illnesses and that all GPs should have some exposure to psychiatry.
>
> p34: Mental health issues should be part of the NMC Foundation Year 2.
>
> p34: The NHS should review the curriculum content – at all education and training levels – to ensure that medical practitioners are able to undertake appropriate cross-sector working (including within NHS ie primary/secondary boundary) as part of their practice.

7.10 The Department is sympathetic to these recommendations and will discuss them with the health professions regulators and with professional and educational interests. Training and continuous professional development for health professionals increasingly recognises the need to work across sectoral boundaries, especially in community settings and in caring for patients with longer term conditions. However, we will discuss with professional and educational interests what more could be done to promote this kind of cross-boundary working.

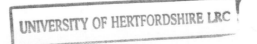

Chapter 8
Information

8.1 As Chapter 4 makes clear, we fully share the Shipman Inquiry's belief that information is the key to enabling NHS employers and PCTs to protect patients from unacceptable professional performance. The Ayling, Neale, Kerr and Haslam cases illustrate the same point: there were enough clues potentially available to indicate serious problems at a much earlier stage. Yet the information was not "joined up" and no effective action was taken. This partly reflects the then prevailing culture[80], in which it was almost unthinkable that health professionals would deliberately set out to harm their patients. But even more, it reflects the fact that NHS organisations did not have the systems and processes to ensure that the relevant information was brought together and critically scrutinised.

8.2 In this chapter, we consider the recommendations of the four inquiries both on the overall systems for storing and giving access to information, and on particular sources of information that could be of value in identifying the warning signals of poor performance.

Information held by individual employers or PCTs

Shipman Inquiry recommendation 33: PCTs should keep a separate file for each individual GP on their lists. That file should hold all material relating to the doctor which could have any possible relevance to clinical governance. If a doctor moves from one PCT to another, the file (or a copy of it) should be sent to the new PCT. It might be helpful if the DoH were to establish national criteria for the content of the files to be kept by PCTs.

Ayling Inquiry para 2.42: We recommend that all NHS Trusts and health care organisations such as deputising services directly employing staff should require them (and particularly part-time staff) to make a formal declaration of any other concurrent employment, not only for obvious health and safety reasons but also to ensure a record is kept of other organisations with an interest in the individual's performance. Failure to make such a declaration should be a disciplinary matter. This requirement should be appropriately adapted for PCTs to be kept informed of other professional employment undertaken by GP.

Para 2.44: We recommend that copies of any written records regarding complaints and concerns and the outcome of these which name an individual practitioner should be placed on that practitioner's personnel file, to be kept for the length of their contract with that organisation. This should be made known to the practitioner concerned.

Kerr/Haslam Inquiry p28: Within 12 months of publication of this Report, the Department of Health should issue guidance as to how and where any disclosure or complaint of abuse by another healthcare professional made to a doctor or nurse should be recorded (if at all) in the patient's medical records, and elsewhere.

Kerr/Haslam Inquiry p32: The Department of Health should convene a working party to consider what information it is necessary to record about complaints in order for them to be of use in clinical governance and the circumstances and form in which it is appropriate to record suspicions.

p33: The Department of Health should clearly state what information can be included in relation to electronic staff records relating to complaints, proven/unproven incidents, disciplinary investigations and findings. Such a record should be established in standard form and, once established, should move with the individual to reduce the risk of staff evading detection of past misdemeanours.

p33: Regulatory bodies (with responsibility for the regulation and discipline of psychiatrists and other mental healthcare professionals) and the Department of Health should be under a clear duty, in the public interest, to share information about disciplinary investigations or other related proceedings. This duty should extend to information known to the regulatory bodies and the Department of Health relating to disciplinary investigations and related proceedings, even if conducted outside the United Kingdom. Consideration should be given to the collection and retention of all information relevant to patient safety, including unsubstantiated complaints, unproven allegations and informal concerns.

8.3 The Department agrees in principle that all healthcare organisations should maintain files for each of their professional employees or (for PCTs) for health professionals performing services to patients for whom they are responsible[xi]. We agree that this "file" – which might be a set of paper files or of interconnected electronic files – should hold all material relating to the quality of the services provided by the individual professional. (Much of the information gathered for clinical governance purposes will relate to the practice or clinical team rather than to the individual; we do not think it would be helpful to duplicate this material in the individual files, but it could be cross-referenced.)

8.4 We recognise the importance of ensuring that PCTs and employers are aware of concurrent employment of health professionals and have made arrangements to share information on concerns, especially where patient safety is at issue. The 2006 Health Act[81] contains an explicit duty on healthcare organisations to share information related specifically to concerns over the possible misuse or diversion of controlled drugs, and related guidance has been issued describing the role of local "networks" coordinated by the Accountable Officer of a lead PCT[82]. **We will discuss with stakeholders the possibility of extending these principles to the sharing of other information relating to potential threats to patient safety.**

8.5 The Department agrees that, if a health professional moves from one organisation to another, the file should with their knowledge be transferred to the new organisation. Similarly, if a professional works regularly for patients of more than one healthcare organisation – for instance, a GP who provides services to patients as a partner of a primary care practice but also has a sessional appointment in a secondary care trust – then a copy of relevant information in the file should be made available to the other PCT/trust, with arrangements for regular updating.

8.6 We agree that the Department, or another central organisation such as NHS Employers, should issue guidance on the content of files to be kept by PCTs and employers, and also on the principles for creating and giving access to records. This will be taken forward in

---

xi There is a particular issue for primary care practitioners who are on the Performers List of one PCT but provide services to patients in another PCT; for instance, under current arrangements, a GP can move to a completely different area but still stay on the Performers List of their original PCT. The principles set out in this section will still apply in these circumstances, but the detailed implementation will be for discussion in the review of the Performers List arrangements described at para 4.35 above.

conjunction with the work on information sharing described in para 6.15 of *Trust, assurance and safety*. There are sensitive issues about the nature of the information that might be stored and about the balance to be struck between the need to protect patients and the human rights of health professionals. For doctors, this work will link with the proposed implementation of the Shipman Inquiry's recommendation for a central database of clinical governance issues (see para 8.7 below) and for the development of the role of the GMC affiliate described in Chapter 3 of *Trust, assurance and safety*.

Information held centrally

Shipman Inquiry recommendation 40: There should be a central database containing information about every doctor working in the UK. This should be accessible to the officers of NHS bodies and to accredited employers in the private sector, as well as to other bodies with a legitimate interest, such as the Healthcare Commission, the GMC, the NCAS and the DoH.

Recommendation 41: The database would contain, or provide links to, information held by the GMC, the Criminal Records Bureau (CRB) and the NHS Counter Fraud and Security Management Service. It would also contain records of disciplinary action by employers, details of list management action by PCTs, any adverse reports following the investigation of a complaint, any adverse findings by a Healthcare Commission panel or by the Healthcare Ombudsman and details of any findings of negligence in a clinical negligence action and settlement of a clinical negligence claim above a pre-determined level of damages. It should also contain certain other information. Doctors would be able to access their own entries to check the accuracy of the information held.

Recommendation 42: Private sector employers should be required to provide relevant information as a condition of registration with the Healthcare Commission. Deputing services should also be required to provide information and should be able to access the database through the relevant PCT.

Recommendation 43: Information about unsubstantiated allegations or concerns should not be included on the central database. Instead, the doctor's entry on the database should be flagged to indicate that confidential information is held by a named NHS body or by the CRB [Criminal Records Bureau] or the GMC or the NHS Counter Fraud and Security Management Service. Questions of access to that information would depend on who was asking for it and for what purpose and would have to be determined at a high level.

Kerr/Haslam Inquiry p31: PALS and complaints staff should be actively linked into a clinical governance and information sharing network with regular access to data on performance issues drawn from such things as claims, patient satisfaction surveys, audit and peer review.

Kerr/Haslam Inquiry p32: In line with the recommendations of the Shipman Inquiry, a centralised database [should] be set up which is capable of recording a range of information about the performance of individual doctors.

Kerr/Haslam Inquiry p33: The Department of Health should clearly state what information can be included in relation to electronic staff records relating to complaints, proven/unproven incidents, disciplinary investigations and findings. Such a record should be established in standard form and, once established, should move with the individual to reduce the risk of staff evading detection of past misdemeanours. The Department of Health should consider whether or not, and if so how and in what circumstances, any such information should be transferable between the NHS and the private sector.

8.7 The case for a central database of information, to protect patients by promoting the sharing of certain information on professional performance between healthcare organisations, is examined in *Good doctors, safer patients*[83]. In the light of the response to consultation, the Government agrees that for doctors the GMC's Medical Register should be the key national list of doctors entitled to practise in the United Kingdom and should contain tiers of information about each doctor and their standard of practice. The Department will discuss with the GMC and other stakeholders how the Register could be developed for this purpose; and will invite the regulators for the other professions to consider whether similar arrangements would be appropriate. Further details are in *Trust, assurance and safety* at paras 6.8-6.12.

Particular categories of information

Practice profiling

8.8 "Practice profiles" are sets of indicators which can be used to assess the quality of the services provided by primary care practices in relation to the healthcare needs of the population they serve. Typically, practice profiles bring together

- demographic data about the practice population

- prescribing data

- other clinical information derived from the practice computer system

- key results of patient satisfaction surveys

and the results can be shown either as a comparison across all the practices in the PCT or as trends over time. Good examples have been developed in a number of PCTs, including Tower Hamlets[84] and Croydon[85].

8.9 *Good doctors, safer patients* recommended that

Further work should be undertaken with the [RCGP] to examine the wider role of practice profiling and the use of other routinely available data in the assurance and improvement of the quality of services delivered in primary care.[86]

The Government agrees and will progress this work with the RCGP, with leading practitioners in PCTs, and with other stakeholders. The intention should be to make the maximum use of existing information streams and to feed back results in a way that is most useful to practices and to commissioners, rather than to impose a new burden of information collection.

Prescribing information

> Shipman Inquiry recommendation 20: Steps should be taken to ensure that every prescription generated by a GP can be accurately attributed to an individual doctor. Only then will the data resulting from the monitoring of prescribing information constitute a reliable clinical governance tool.
>
> Recommendation 21: Regular monitoring of GPs' prescribing should be undertaken by PCTs. Special attention should be paid to the prescribing of controlled drugs by GPs. Doctors who have had a problem of drug misuse in the past or who are suspected of having a current problem should be subjected to particularly close scrutiny. When a restriction is placed on a doctor's prescribing powers, this information must be made available (preferably by electronic means) to those who need to know, particularly pharmacists.

8.10 Work is already in hand to implement these recommendations, following the similar recommendations in the Shipman Inquiry's fourth report[87].

8.11 Even when prescribing data is accurately allocated to the individual doctor responsible for the prescribing decision, it is not easy to interpret; even apparently anomalous prescribing patterns can have a perfectly legitimate explanation. As part of the previous work on practice profiling and as recommended in *Good doctors, safer patients*, **the Government will invite the RCGP to work with the Prescribing Support Unit (now part of the NHS Information Centre) on the way in which prescribing data can be used to assure the quality of GP services**.

Mortality data

> Shipman Inquiry recommendation 22: The Department of Health should make provision for a national system for monitoring GP patient mortality rates. The system should be supported by a well organised, consistent and objective means of investigating those cases where a GP's patient mortality rates signal as being above the norm.
>
> Recommendation 23: Every GP practice should keep a death register in which the particulars of the deaths of patients of the practice should be recorded for use in audit and for other purposes.

8.12 The NHS Information Centre, in collaboration with the Office of National Statistics (ONS), has now developed a Primary Care Mortality Database linking mortality data to primary care practices. The database can by accessed by PCT staff subject to signing the ONS confidentiality declaration. However, earlier work by the Department suggests that practice-level mortality data on its own may have only limited use for clinical governance purposes. A similar pilot study in Northern Ireland[88] showed that it was feasible to identify statistical "outliers" but found that in each case there was a reasonable explanation for the unusual mortality rates found. The issues are not straightforward and **we will explore further with stakeholders the potential use of practice-level mortality data as a clinical governance tool**.

8.13 We agree in principle that it would be helpful for all practices to keep a register of the deaths of their registered patients, including those who die in secondary care, for use in local clinical audit. Some individual GPs have developed impressive systems of this nature but their use is not yet widespread. *Good doctors, safer patients* recommended that

> The NHS should support the routine monitoring of significant events in general practice through the contracts of general practitioners, further developing and piloting a national system for death monitoring as part of a wider clinical quality assurance framework in general practice.[89]

This links with the outline proposals which we are announcing in *Learning from tragedy – keeping patients safe* (see para 1.12) for a new approach to validating and using the information from death certificates, responding to recommendations in the Shipman Inquiry's third report. The Government will shortly be publishing a consultation document with further detail on the proposed arrangements. **As part of this consultation we will discuss with the RCGP, GP interests and other stakeholders the potential use of significant event monitoring, including the monitoring of deaths**.

Information on clinical negligence claims

> Shipman Inquiry recommendation 44: GPs should be required to disclose to the relevant PCT the fact that a clinical negligence claim has been brought against them, the gist of the allegation made and, when the time comes, the outcome of the claim.

8.14 The Department has discussed this proposal with the NHS Litigation Authority and with the Medical Defence Unions (MDUs). Although at first sight clinical negligence claims might also seem a useful indication of possible issues with the quality of GPs' or other doctors' clinical care, there are significant difficulties:

- since the 1999 reforms to the clinical negligence process, MDU experience is that about 70% of claims are discontinued, usually because initial inquiries have shown that no negligence was involved;

- the majority of the remaining cases are settled out of court, but without any admission of liability on the doctor's part. Requiring GPs to notify only settled cases to their PCT might act as a disincentive to settling claims out of court, increasing the trauma to patients and doctors and the likely cost to public funds;

- there is often a considerable time lag in bringing clinical negligence cases. As a result, where cases are taken to the end of a process and a finding made against the doctor, many years may have elapsed since the original event and the fact that an adverse finding has been made may not be any reflection on the current quality of care of the doctor.

In the light of these difficulties, it is clear that clinical negligence claims should be reported to PCTs (if at all) only in order to maintain a broad overview of the pattern of complaints and concerns about the doctor and not with any presumption that the rate of claims is a reliable indicator of the quality of the doctor's practice. **We will discuss these issues further with relevant stakeholders in parallel with the similar recommendations from the Shipman Inquiry on notifying complaints** (see para 5.25) **and concerns from fellow professionals** (see para 5.34).

Information for patients and the general public

Information on health professionals

Shipman Inquiry recommendation 45: The GMC should adopt a policy of tiered disclosure to apply to all persons seeking information about a doctor.

Recommendation 46: The first tier should relate to information which is relevant to the doctor's current registration status, together with certain information about his/her past FTP [fitness to practise] history. First tier information should be posted on the GMC website and should also be disclosed to anyone who requests information about the doctor's registration. The periods of time for which information should remain at the first tier should depend on the nature of the information. When the relevant period expires, the information should be removed from the website. It should be replaced by a note indicating that there is further information which can be obtained by telephoning the GMC. That information should then be available at the second tier.

Recommendation 47: Disclosure of information at the second tier should be made to any person who makes a request about a doctor's FTP history. All information which has at any time been in the public domain should remain available to enquirers at the second tier for as long as the doctor remains on the register.

8.15 The Department agrees with the principles underlying these recommendations and will discuss them further with the health professions regulators, including the CHRE, and with professional and patient interests. We understand that the GMC has already implemented a form of tiered disclosure after widespread consultation on similar proposals to those in the Shipman Inquiry's report.

Shipman Inquiry recommendation 48: In all cases where a GP's registration is subject to conditions, or where s/he has resumed practice after a period of suspension or erasure, patients of any practice in which the GP works should be told. A letter of explanation, which has been approved by the PCT, should be sent to all patients. Patients should have the opportunity to refuse to be treated by a doctor who is subject to conditions or who has previously been subject to an order for suspension or erasure.

8.16 The Department is sympathetic to the intention behind this recommendation. At the same time, a balance needs to be struck between the public interest in helping to rehabilitate a health professional who is subject to restrictions or who is returning from suspension or erasure from the professional register, and the legitimate right of patients to know the position. *Trust, assurance and safety* emphasises at paras 4.21-25 the importance of ensuring that rehabilitation is available to health professionals who have made honest mistakes, or who have been suffering from stress or other health problems, but who could still have a valuable contribution to make if their return to work, can be sensitively handled. The issues are not straightforward and we will discuss further with NHS, professional and patient groups the best way of taking these proposals forward.

Information on treatments and on treatment outcomes

> Kerr/Haslam Inquiry p24: In relation to such identified "new or unorthodox treatments", patients should be given written explanations of the treatments, and why their use is appropriate.
>
> p28: Mental health services should provide routine information to patients attending appointments on what to expect from a consultation with a mental health professional. This should apply to consultations in all settings, including home visits.
>
> p36: The Mental Health Trusts, together with the Primary Care Trusts, should draw up and distribute patient information leaflets, so that patients referred by their General Practitioners to the care of a consultant psychiatrist can better understand what to expect, and the circumstances if any in which the patient can expect to receive any physical examination or treatment from the psychiatrist [further detail at Annex F]

8.17 The Government agrees that patients should be fully informed about treatment options or recommendations, and should as far as possible take part in an informed dialogue with their clinicians on the choice of treatment. At the very least, patients must have sufficient information to give informed consent to *any* treatment and that this is particularly important for "new or unorthodox" treatments, ie in this context treatments which are not part of the standard repertoire of treatments for the condition concerned. **The Government will ensure that the need for adequate information to patients is covered in the guidance described at para 4.43 above, relating to the role of clinical governance committees in sanctioning such treatments.**

8.18 For more conventional therapies it is reasonable to expect that the GP or other health professional referring a patient for specialist treatment will describe in broad terms the likely assessment and therapeutic purpose of the consultation. Many GPs and hospital outpatient clinics will reinforce this by providing information leaflets.

8.19 The Department of Health is developing an Information Accreditation Scheme[90] which will raise the general standard of such information and help the public to find reliable sources of information. We are also testing out a set of "questions to ask" to help people, including those in disadvantaged groups, to prepare for consultations and empower them to ask appropriate questions.

> Neale Inquiry recommendation 15: Patients should receive copies of letters sent to and from their general practitioners and in the template of the letter sent to all patients, the doctor should confirm, "I have discussed the condition and treatment with the patient."
>
> Neale Inquiry recommendation 16: In the patient's copy of the discharge letter the doctor should complete as appropriate, that, "the procedure went to plan/had the following complications… This has/has not been discussed with the patient".
>
> Neale Inquiry recommendation 17: If a consultant has not performed a procedure or part of a procedure himself he should legibly identify who did and whether it was under supervision. Patients should know who operated on them.

8.20 The Government agrees that patients should have the opportunity to receive copies of letters between their GPs and specialist clinicians. These letters should not be a substitute for information given face to face at consultations; written information to patients should reinforce the information they have already been given in consultations, which will include the patient's condition, the recommended treatment for which they are being referred (for referral letters), and the outcomes of treatment (for discharge letters).

8.21 The Department of Health announced its initiative "Copying letters to patients" in the NHS plan in 2000 and issued further guidance on implementing the initiative in 2003[91]. The guidance includes suggested templates setting out the information that can be included in letters, including items like diagnosis, management recommendations and the results of investigations as well as information given to patients. The guidance makes clear that patients should be asked whether they wish to receive copies of letters and that their decision should be recorded in local systems.

8.22 The Government agrees that patients should be told, at least in broad terms, about the outcomes of treatment. Professional guidance from the GMC and from the medical defence organisations encourages doctors to be open with their patients about complications or adverse events, but the level of detail of the information to be disclosed must ultimately be for the professional judgement of the clinician and we would not want to be prescriptive in this sensitive area.

Chapter 9
Summary of Action Programme

9.1 In conjunction with the action set out in *Trust, assurance and safety* this response sets out a comprehensive programme of action to respond to the issues raised by the Shipman, Ayling, Neale and Kerr/Haslam inquiries. Our aim is to ensure that problems with the behaviour or competence of health professionals are quickly identified and rigorously investigated and that action is taken to protect patients and – wherever possible – help the individual to remedy the identified problems. And we wish to do so in a way that works with the grain of existing NHS clinical governance systems and that supports and encourages the vast majority of health professionals who are seeking to give the best possible care to their patients.

9.2 This chapter summarises the main actions described in this response. Some are already under way; others will be put in hand as soon as possible. The final section of the chapter describes how we will take forward this ambitious work programme in partnership with the many interested parties, including patient and voluntary organisations, NHS management, professional organisations, and the professional and healthcare regulators.

Recruitment and screening processes

9.3 Guidance in this area is issued by NHS Employers, part of the NHS Confederation, and has already been updated to meet some of the Neale recommendations. The Government:

* will consider the best way of using the new approach to regulation set out in the recent consultation paper *The future regulation of health and social care in England* to promote best practice in this area

* has asked NHS Employers to ensure that future updates of its guidance take account of all the Neale Inquiry's recommendations.

Clinical governance

9.4 Chapter 4 sets out the Government's belief that action to respond to the central concerns of the four inquiries should build on and strengthen existing clinical governance processes, not replace them. This is fully consistent with the approach taken by the Government to improving the management of controlled drugs in response to the Shipman Inquiry's fourth report and with the proposed reform of procedures for scrutinising death certificates outlined in a companion paper published today.

9.5 The Government fully accepts that more is needed to strengthen clinical governance processes and to embed the culture of clinical governance in every NHS organisation. Among other changes, the Government:

● will consider how the statutory "duty of quality" on all NHS organisations can be strengthened to underline the duty to investigate and learn from complaints and medical errors;

● will issue further guidance on the investigation of complaints and concerns, including overlapping investigations involving the police or professional regulators;

● as part of this work, has asked the Commission for Healthcare Regulatory Excellence (CHRE) to lead a project to define the standards for local investigations which would enable their findings to be used by professional regulators, and to determine the thresholds at which concerns should be referred on to the regulators;

● will consider extending the role of the National Clinical Assessment Service (NCAS) to provide advice to healthcare organisations for health professionals other than doctors and dentists;

● in primary care, will consider how the accountability of GPs to their PCT can be further strengthened, as proposed in *Good doctors, safer patients*, including clarifying the right of access of PCTs to patients' medical records when needed in the course of an investigation; and

● will review the Performers List arrangements, including considering the Shipman Inquiry's proposal for a range of lesser sanctions as an alternative to suspended or removing primary care professionals from the list.

Complaints and concerns

9.6 The Government agrees that complaints (from patients or their representatives) and concerns (from fellow professionals) can provide vital information in identifying potential risks to patient safety, as well as more generally indicating how services can be improved. There have already been major developments in this area in recent years. Chapter 5 summarises recent changes and refers to the major review of the complaints systems for both health and social care launched by the Department in 2006 following a commitment in the community services White Paper *Our health, our care, our say*. As part of this programme the Government

● will shortly issue a consultation paper with proposals for a new complaints system;

● as part of this consultation, will consult on possible developments to the current national standards relating to the handling of complaints in health and social care;

● will work with stakeholders on a set of common standards for the initial handling of complaints to ensure that, wherever patients first direct a complaint, it is speedily transferred to the most appropriate organisation;

● subject to consultation, will amend the complaints regulations to enable patients or their representatives to make complaints about treatment in general medical practice directly to their PCT, and to require PCTs to take an overview of all such complaints even where they are handled by the practice;

- is supporting complaints handlers in general practice by setting up networks for mutual support;

- will ensure that all organisations providing services to NHS patients have clear policies setting out how staff can raise concerns;

- will explore the potential role of SHAs or PCTs in receiving concerns where the member of staff feels unable to go to their own employer; and

- will explore with professional regulators and universities how the duty on health professionals to report concerns about fellow professionals can be further emphasised, especially in undergraduate education.

Boundary transgressions and particular issues in mental health services

9.7 Chapter 6 considers the recommendations in the Kerr/Haslam and Ayling inquiries about the failure of health organisations to take seriously allegations of sexual assault on female patients. Since the period covered by the two inquiries there is now much more awareness of the issue of sexual or other abuse by health professionals, thanks in no small measure to the courage of the victims in coming forward and bringing their experiences into the public domain. But further work is needed to both to develop guidance and to ensure that all staff working in the NHS are fully aware of the issues.

9.8 The Department has commissioned CHRE to carry out a major exercise which will among other things

- develop detailed and comprehensive guidance for health professionals and their regulators on the proper boundaries which professionals should maintain between themselves and their patients;

- develop guidance for NHS and other healthcare employers on how to prevent, detect and investigate boundary violations; and

- develop a common approach to educational standards on boundary issues for adoption into training programmes for professionals.

9.9 Patients in mental health settings are particularly vulnerable to potential boundary violations. Chapter 7 discusses the recommendations relating to this particular group of patients in the Kerr/Haslam report. In general, the Government believes that the principles of clinical governance which apply in other settings are equally relevant to mental health, but agrees that special attention may be needed to issues such as

- the use of information disclosed in the therapeutic setting;

- advocacy support for patients wishing to make a complaint; and

- training in mental health issues for health professionals.

The Government will discuss further with stakeholders and issue further guidance as needed.

Information

9.10 All four inquiries stress the key role of information in identifying potential problems of professional behaviour or competence and alerting healthcare organisations to the need to take action to protect patients. Often, relevant information is held by different organisations or different parts of one organisation, and it is only by "triangulating" this information that the true extent of problems are revealed. At the same time, sharing information between organisations, especially "soft" information such as unsubstantiated complaints or concerns, raises difficult issues about confidentiality and the human rights of individual professionals.

9.11 Chapter 8 reviews the recommendations in this area from the four inquiries and from *Good doctors, safer patients*. The Government will

- issue or commission guidance on the content of files kept by healthcare organisations about health professionals employed by or in contract with them and about the circumstances in which such information can be shared with other organisations;

- discuss with stakeholders the possibility of extending, to performance issues more generally, the concept in the 2006 Health Act of a statutory duty to share information where needed to protect the public;

- progress, with the Royal College of General Practitioners (RCGP) and other stakeholders, work on indicators of the quality of services provided by primary care practices ("practice profiling"), including the use of prescribing indicators and information on mortality; and

- discuss further the proposal from the Shipman Inquiry that GPs should be required to disclose all clinical negligence claims to their PCT.

9.12 In addition, as announced in *Trust, assurance and safety*, the Government has accepted the recommendations in the CMO's review that the GMC register should become the main source of information on doctors' registration status and on any disciplinary action, including "recorded concerns" (a formal note of a concern over professional conduct or competency which the doctor has accepted but is not regarded as significant enough to require referral to the GMC's central fitness to practise proceedings). There will be "tiered" access to this information, with some parts of the information base generally available and other parts available only to NHS and other accredited healthcare employers.

Taking the action forward

9.13 As already noted, the action stemming from this document and from *Trust, assurance and safety* should be seen as a single programme of action to ensure patient safety, and to reassure the public that the NHS has learnt from the lessons of the Shipman and other high-profile cases. Although the broad thrust is clear, many issues of detail remain which the Department of Health will need to discuss with patient, NHS and professional groups and with the health professions regulators. The Department will

- in due course publish an integrated action plan setting out a timetable for all the action envisaged in the two documents; and

- establish a national advisory group with all relevant stakeholders to advise the Department on implementation.

References

1. Shipman Inquiry *Safeguarding patients: lessons from the past – proposals for the future*, Cm 6394 (TSO, December 2004)

2. Shipman Inquiry *Death certification and the investigation of deaths by coroners*, Cm 5854 (TSO, July 2003)

3. Shipman Inquiry *The regulation of controlled drugs in the community*, Cm 6249 (TSO, July 2004)

4. Ayling Inquiry *Independent investigation into how the NHS handled allegations about the conduct of Clifford Ayling*, Cm 6298 (TSO, September 2004)

5. Neale Inquiry *Independent investigation into how the NHS handled allegations about the conduct of Richard Neale*, Cm 6315 (TSO, September 2004)

6. Kerr/Haslam Inquiry *Independent investigation into how the NHS handled allegations about the conduct of William Kerr and Michael Haslam*, Cm 6640 (TSO, July 2005)

7. Kerr/Haslam Inquiry page 36: "If not already appointed, a multidisciplinary committee should be established to collate, consider and report on the recommendations made in this Report, in the Shipman Report, the Neale Report, the Ayling Report, and the Peter Green Report, insofar as those reports, and the recommendations made in them relate to the common theme of handling concerns and complaints, and to patient protection"

8. *Good doctors, safer patients: proposals to strengthen the system to assure and improve the performance of doctors and to protect the safety of patients – a report by the Chief Medical Officer* (Department of Health, July 2006)

9. *The regulation of the non-medical healthcare professions: a review by the Department of Health* (Department of Health, July 2006)

10. *Trust, assurance and safety – the regulation of health professionals in the 21st century* (Department of Health, February 2007)

11. *Creating a patient-led NHS – delivering the NHS improvement plan* (Department of Health, March 2005)

12. *Commissioning for a patient-led NHS* (Department of Health, July 2005)

13. *Learning from tragedy – keeping patients safe* (Department of Health, February 2007)

14. *A first class service: quality in the new NHS* (Department of Health, July 1998)

15. *National standards, local action* (Department of Health, July 2004)

16. Bristol Royal Infirmary Inquiry *Learning from Bristol*, Cm 5207 (TSO, July 2001); *Learning from Bristol: the Department of Health's response to the report of the public inquiry into children's heart surgery at Bristol Royal Infirmary 1984-1995*, Cm 5363 (TSO, January 2002)

17. *Independent health care: national minimum standards and regulations* (Department of Health, February 2002)

18. *The future regulation of health and adult social care in England* (Department of Health, December 2006)

19. *The new NHS: modern, dependable* (Department of Health, December 1997)

20. *A first class service: quality in the new NHS* (Department of Health, July 1998)

21. *Steps towards clinical governance* (Department of Health, January 1999); *Clinical governance – a practical guide for primary care teams* (Department of Health, January 1999)

22. Health and Social Care Act 2001

23. *Maintaining high professional standards in the modern NHS* (Department of Health, February 2005)

24. ACAS *Code of Practice 1: Disciplinary and grievance procedures* (TSO, 2003)

25. *Supporting doctors, protecting patients* (Department of Health, November 1999)

26. *Assuring the quality of medical practice: implementing 'Supporting doctors, protecting patients'* (Department of Health, January 2001)

27. *An organisation with a memory* (Department of Health, June 2000)

28. *Building a safer NHS for patients: implementing 'An organisation with a memory'* (Department of Health, June 2001)

29. *A safer place for patients: learning to improve patient safety* (National Audit Office, November 2005)

30. *Safety first* (Department of Health, December 2006)

31. *Better information, better choices, better health* (Department of Health, December 2004)

32. *The expert patient: a new approach to chronic disease management for the 21st century* (Department of Health, June 2004)

33. Section 11 of the Health and Social Care Act 2001

34. *A stronger local voice* (Department of Health, July 2006)

35. *Government response to 'A stronger local voice'* (Department of Health, December 2006)

36. NHS Redress Act 2006

37. *Health reform in England: update and next steps* (Department of Health, December 2005)

38. *Our health, our care, our say: a new direction for community services* (Department of Health, January 2006)

39. *Keeping it personal: clinical case for change* (Department of Health, February 2007)

40. Better Regulation Task Force *Principles of good regulation* (Cabinet Office 1997, revised 2000 and 2003)

41. Hampton Review *Reducing administrative burdens: effective inspection and enforcement* (HM Treasury March 2005)

42. See reference 1, pages 106–9

43. See the website for the NHS electronic staff record at http://www.esrsolution.co.uk/

44. *Safer recruitment: a guide for NHS employers* (NHS Employers, January 2007)

45. *NHS contracts for 2007/2008 and guidance on the NHS contract for acute hospital services 2007/08* (Department of Health, December 2006)

46. See reference 3, recommendation 6

47. *Safer management of controlled drugs: the government response to the Fourth Report of the Shipman Inquiry*, Cm 6343 (TSO, December 2004)

48. *Achieving improvements through clinical governance: a progress report on implementation by NHS Trusts* (National Audit Office, September 2003)

49. *Improving quality and safety – progress in implementing clinical governance in primary care* (National Audit Office, January 2007)

50. *Primary care dental services: clinical governance framework* (NHS Primary Care Contracting, May 2006)

51. Reference 8, recommendations 2 and 3

52. See Section 45 of the Health and Social Care (Community Health and Standards) Act 2003

53. See reference 36, section 10(3)

54. *Local GP performance procedures*, available on the NCAS website www.ncas.npsa.nhs.uk/toolkit

55. Department of Health/National Patient Safety Agency *Handling concerns about the performance of healthcare professionals: principles of good practice* (Department of Health, September 2006)

56. *Memorandum of understanding: Investigating patient safety incidents involving unexpected death or serious untoward harm* (Association of Chief Police Officers, Department of Health, and Health and Safety Executive, February 2006)

57. *Information sharing protocol between the General Medical Council, the Nursing and Midwifery Council, the Association of Chief Police Officers and the Crown Prosecution Service* (July 2006)

58. See reference 38 para 7.22-23

59. *Practice based commissioning: practical implementation* (Department of Health, November 2006)

60. Reference 8. recommendation 36

61. See reference 10. para [ ] {page 35, standards for relicensure]

62. See *Confidentiality and disclosure of information: GMS, PMS and APMS code of practice* (Department of Health [add date]), especially paras 30–2

63. Sheffield School of Health and Related Research *GPs convicted of criminal offences: the primary care trust response* (ScHARR November 2005) – available on request from the Department of Health, Quality and Standards Directorate

64. See reference 10, para [3.17]

65. Family Health Services Appeal Authority Annual Report 2004–05 (July 2005)

66. The consultation is at www.nice.org.uk/page.aspx?o=ipmethodsguide

67. National Health Service (Complaints) Regulations 2004 (SI 2004 No1768)

68. National Health Service (Complaints) Amendment Regulations (SI 2006 No 2084)

69. *Independent health care: national minimum standards and regulations* (Department of Health, February 2002)

70. MORI survey quoted on p75 of *Making amends – clinical negligence reform* (Department of Health, October 2003)

71. *Handling complaints in the NHS – good practice toolkit for local resolution* (Department of Health, updated April 2004)

72. National Health Services (General Medical Services Contracts) Regulations 2004 (SI 2004 no 906)

73. NCAS *Concerned about the performance of a colleague?* (March 2004, updated 2006)

74. See their website at www.popan.org.uk

75. Based on a review of 14 research papers cited in Witness, *A comparison of UK health regulators' guidance on professional boundaries* (CHRE, January 2005)

76. See *Practitioner-client relationships and the prevention of abuse* (Nursing and Midwifery Council 2002); *Maintaining boundaries* (GMC, November 2006). Other guidance is summarised in reference Error! Bookmark not defined.

77. *Guidance on the role and effective use of chaperones in primary and community care* (National Clinical Governance Support Team, June 2006 (updated October 2005))

78. *No secrets: guidance on developing and implementing multi-agency policies and procedures to protect vulnerable adults from abuse* (Department of Health and Home Office, March 2000) especially paras 3.10 and 5.2

79. *Protection of vulnerable adults scheme – a practical guide* (Department of Health, updated May 2006)

80. See for instance para 82 of the summary of the Shipman Inquiry's fifth report and para 4.3 of the report of the Ayling Inquiry.

81. Health Act 2006, Part 3, Chapter 1, Supervision of management and use of controlled drugs

82. *Safer management of controlled drugs: guidance on strengthened governance arrangements* (Department of Health, updated January 2007)

83. Reference 8, recommendation 38

84. On the Primary Care Contracting website at http://www.pcc.nhs.uk/uploads/balanced_score_card_dec_06/balanced_scorecard_final.pdf

85. Private communication from Dr Tim Crayford, Croydon PCT

86. Reference 8, recommendation 34

87. See references 3 and 47

88.   Mohammed et al "A practical method for monitoring general practice mortality in the UK: findings from a pilot study in a health board of Northern Ireland", *British Journal of General Practice* 55 670 (September 2005)

89.   Reference 8, recommendation 34

90.   See reference 31, Chapter 2

91.   *Copying letters to patients: good practice guidelines* (Department of Health, April 2003)

List of abbreviations

CHAI	Commission for Healthcare Audit and Inspection (now the Healthcare Commission)
CHRE	Council for Healthcare Regulatory Excellence
CMO	Chief Medical Officer
CPD	Continuous Professional Development
CRB	Criminal Records Bureau
FHSAA	Family Health Services Appeal Authority
FTP	Fitness to practise
GMC	General Medical Council
ICAS	Independent Complaints Advisory Service
LMC	Local Medical Committee
MDU	Medical Defense Union
MHRA	Medicines and Healthcare products Regulatory Agency
MOU	Memorandum of Understanding
NAO	National Audit Office
NCAS	National Clinical Assessment Service (formerly the National Clinical Assessment Authority, NCAA)
NICE	National Institute of Health and Clinical Excellence
NIMHE	National Institute for Mental Health in England
NPSA	National Patient Safety Agency
NRLS	National Reporting and Learning System
PALS	Patient Liaison Service
PBC	Practice-based commissioning (or Practice-based commissioner)
PCT	Primary care trust
PSAT	Patient safety action team
RCGP	Royal College of General Practitioners
ScHARR	Sheffield School for Health and Related Research
SHA	Strategic health authority

Annex A
Terms of reference of the inquiries

Shipman Inquiry

(a)   After receiving the existing evidence and hearing such further evidence as necessary, to consider the extent of Harold Shipman's unlawful activities;

(b)   To enquire into the actions of the statutory bodies, authorities, other organisations and responsible individuals concerned in the procedures and investigations which followed the deaths of those of Harold Shipman's patients who died in unlawful or suspicious circumstances;

(c)   By reference to the case of Harold Shipman to enquire into the performance of the functions of those statutory bodies, authorities, other organisations and individuals with responsibility for monitoring primary care provision and the use of controlled drugs; and

(d)   Following those enquiries, to recommend what steps, if any, should be taken to protect patients in the future, and to report its findings to the Secretary of State for the Home Department and to the Secretary of State for Health.

The "three inquiries"

The terms of reference for the three inquiries were almost identical, apart from the details of the doctors concerned and the periods over which the alleged offences were committed. The terms of reference for the Ayling Inquiry were as follows:

The overall purpose of the Inquiry is:

1.   To assess the appropriateness and effectiveness of the procedures operated in the local health services

   (a) for enabling health service users to raise issues of legitimate concern relating to the conduct of health service employees and professionals;

   (b) for ensuring that such complaints are effectively considered; and

   (c) for ensuring that appropriate remedial action is taken in the particular case and generally; and

2.   To make such recommendations as are appropriate for the revision and improvement of the procedures referred to above.

The Inquiry is asked:

- To identify the procedures in place during the period 1971-2000 within the local health services to enable members of the public and other health service users to raise concerns or complaints concerning the actions and conduct of health service professionals in their professional capacity.

- To document and establish the nature of and chronology of the concerns or complaints raised concerning the appointment, practice and conduct of Dr Clifford Ayling, a former GP from Kent, during this period.

- To investigate the actions which were taken for the purpose of (a) considering the concerns and complaints that were raised; (b) providing remedial action in relation to them; and (c) ensuring that the opportunities for any similar future misconduct were removed.

- To investigate cultural or other organisational factors within the local health services, which impeded or prevented appropriate investigation and action.

- To assess and draw conclusions as to the effectiveness of the policies and procedures in place.

- To make recommendations, informed by this case, as to improvements which should be made to the policies and procedures which are now in place within the health service (taking into account the changes in procedure since the events in question).

- To provide a full report on these matters to the Secretary of State for Health for publication by him.

Annex B
Terms of reference for the reviews of medical and non-medical regulation

Review of medical regulation

To provide a report to ministers setting out my advice on further measures that are necessary to:

- strengthen procedures for assuring the safety of patients in situations where a doctor's performance or conduct pose a risk to patient safety or the effective functioning of services;

- ensure the operation of an effective system of revalidation;

- modify the role, structure and functions of the General Medical Council.

Review of non-medical regulation

To consider and advise the Secretary of State about the measures needed to:

- strengthen procedures for ensuring that the performance or conduct of non-medical health professionals and other health service staff does not pose a threat to patient safety or the effective functioning of services, particularly focusing on the effective and fair operation of fitness to practise procedures;

- ensure the operation of effective systems of continuing professional development and appraisal for non-medical health care staff and make progress towards revalidation where appropriate;

- ensure the effective regulation of healthcare staff working in new roles within the healthcare sector and of other staff in regular contact with patients;

and in the light of these to consider and recommend any changes needed to the role, structure, functions and a number of regulators of non-medical healthcare professional staff.

Annex C
Recommendations of the Shipman Inquiry's fifth report

Rec	Inquiry recommendation	Government response	
		Para	**Response**
1a	I endorse the provision contained in the draft National Health Service (Complaints) Regulations (the draft Complaints Regulations), whereby patients and their representatives who wish to make a complaint against a general practitioner (GP) will be permitted to choose whether to lodge that complaint with the GP practice concerned or with the local PCT.	5.25	Accept subject to further consultation.
1b	... I also endorse the provision extending the time limit for complaining from six to twelve months.		Accept.
2	Steps should be taken to improve the standard of complaints handling by GP practices.	5.29–30	Accept – action already in hand.
3	Draft regulation 30 of the draft Complaints Regulations, which would require GP practices to provide primary care trusts (PCTs) with limited information about complaints received by the practice at intervals to be specified by the PCT, should be amended. The GP practice should be required to report all complaints to the PCT within, say, two working days of their receipt. The report should contain the original letter of complaint or, if the complaint was made orally, the practice's record of the complaint. The PCT should log the complaint for clinical governance purposes and, if it considers that the complaint raises clinical governance issues, it should 'call in' the complaint for investigation.	5.25	Accept in principle, subject to consultation.
4	There should be statutory recognition of the importance of the proper investigation of complaints to the processes of clinical governance and of monitoring the quality of health care.	4.13–14	Accept.

Rec	Inquiry recommendation	Government response	
		Para	Response
5	On receipt by a PCT of a complaint about a GP, a 'triage' (the first triage) of the complaint should be conducted by a member of the PCT's staff who is appropriately experienced and has access to relevant clinical advice. The object of the first triage should be to assess whether the complaint arises from a purely private grievance or raises clinical governance issues.	5.14	We will discuss with stakeholders, as part of the formal consultation on a revised complaints framework, how to promote best practice in identifying the most serious complaints.
6	'Private grievance complaints' should be dealt with by appropriately trained PCT staff. The objectives in dealing with such complaints should be the satisfaction of the patient and, where possible, restoration of the relationship of trust and confidence between doctor and patient.	5.14–15	In general the government believes that complaints not involving broader issues of patient safety should where possible be resolved by the GP practice. We accept that on occasion an element of mediation by the PCT may be needed.
7a	'Clinical governance complaints' should be investigated [by the PCT] with the dual objectives of patient protection satisfaction and fairness to doctors.	5.14–15	Agree.
7b	'Clinical governance complaints' ... should be referred for a further triage (the second triage) to a small group comprising two or three people – for example, the Medical Director or Clinical Governance Lead, a senior non medical officer of the PCT and a lay member of the PCT board. The object of the second triage should be to decide whether the complaint is to be investigated by or on behalf of the PCT or whether it should instead be referred to some other body, such as the police, the General Medical Council (GMC) or the national Clinical Assessment Authority (NCAA).	4.20–24	Agree that early decision needed on how potential concurrent investigations should be handled. Proposed membership of triage group is consistent with current (NCAS) advice but Government does wish to be too prescriptive on this point.
8	The investigation of 'clinical governance complaints' should not be undertaken by PCT staff. Instead, groups of PCTs should set up joint teams of investigators, who should be properly trained in the techniques of investigation and should adopt an objective and analytical approach, keeping their minds open to all possibilities.	4.34	The Government accepts that this is a useful model which some PCTs have used to good effect, but does not intend to be prescriptive on this point. We will seek further views in consultation.

Rec	Inquiry recommendation	Government response	
		Para	Response
9	All 'clinical governance complaints' (save those which do not involve serious issues of patient safety and where the underlying facts giving rise to the complaint are clear and undisputed) should be referred to the inter-PCT investigation team. The objective of the investigation should be to reach a conclusion as to what happened and to set out the evidence and conclusions in a report which should go to the PCT with responsibility for the doctor. If the investigators are unable to reach a conclusion about what happened because there is an unresolved conflict of evidence, they should say so in their report.	4.15	Agree importance of objective investigation by properly trained investigators. This is consistent with existing DH and NCAS guidance. Further development of guidance in relation to the investigation of complaints will be subject to formal consultation on a revised complaints framework.
10a	On receipt of the report, the PCT group which carried out the second triage should consider what action to take. It might be appropriate to refer the matter to another body, such as the GMC or the NCAA. Alternatively, it might be appropriate for the PCT to take action itself, e.g. by invoking its list management powers.	4.16	Agree need for fair and transparent decision making process, independent of original investigation. This is consistent with existing DH and NCAS guidance. Referral to NCAS for advice or assessment, or to the professional regulator, are options to be considered. For doctors, the GMC affiliate should also be consulted.
10b	If the report of the investigation team is inconclusive, because of a conflict of evidence, the case should be referred to the Commission for Healthcare Audit and Inspection (now known as the Healthcare Commission), under a power which should be included in the amended draft Complaint Regulations when implemented.		Reject (see below on recommendation 13).
11a	Neither an intention on the part of the complainant to take legal proceedings, nor the fact that such proceedings have begun, should be a bar to the investigation by a NHS body of a complaint.	4.24	Agree, provided further investigation by the NHS body does not prejudice possible legal proceedings.
11b	In circumstances where the NHS body is taking disciplinary proceedings relating to the subject matter of the complaint against the person complained of, a complainant should be entitled to see the report of the investigation on which the disciplinary proceedings are to be based and should not merely be informed that the investigation of his/her complaint is to be deferred or discontinued.	4.24	Agree in principle that information relating to the investigation of the complaint should be available, and will issue guidance on this after further consultation.

Rec	Inquiry recommendation	Government response	
		Para	Response
12	In some circumstances, it may be necessary for a NHS body to defer or discontinue its own investigation of a complaint if the matter is being investigated by the police, a regulatory body, a statutory inquiry or some other process. However, a NHS body should never lose sight of its duty to find out what has happened and to take whatever action is necessary for the protection of the patients of the doctor concerned. It should also provide such information to the complainant as is consistent with the need, if any, for confidentiality in the public interest. The relevant provisions of the draft Complaints Regulations should be amended to reflect these principles.	4.23	Agree.
13	The draft Complaints Regulations, when implemented, should include a power enabling PCTs to refer a complaint to the Health Commission for investigation at any point during the first stage of the complaints procedures. Cases raising difficult or complex issues or involving issues relating to both primary and secondary care might be referred to the Healthcare Commission for investigation at the time of the second triage, or later if the investigation by the inter-PCT investigation team raises more complex issues than had initially been apparent. Referral to the Healthcare Commission should also take place in cases where the inter-PCT investigation team has found that it cannot reach a conclusion because there remain unresolved disputes of fact. The purpose of the referral would be for the Healthcare Commission to carry out any further necessary investigation, and, if appropriate, to set up a panel to hear oral evidence about the facts in dispute and to decide where the truth lay.	4.18–19	Agree may be need to help healthcare organisations with the more complex investigations but do not accept that an automatic referral to Healthcare Commission would be helpful. See para 4.19 of response for fuller discussion.
14	Complaints procedures in the private sector should be aligned as closely as possible with those in the NHS, so that a complainant who does not receive a satisfactory response to his/her complaint can proceed to a second stage of the complaints procedures to be conducted by the Healthcare Commission.	5.17	Agree in principle and will work with the Healthcare Commission and with representatives of the independent and voluntary sectors towards this aim.

Rec	Inquiry recommendation	Government response	
		Para	**Response**
15a	Concerns expressed about a GP by someone other than a patient or patient's representative (e.g. by a fellow healthcare professional) should be dealt with in the same way as patient complaints. Such concerns should be investigated (where necessary) by the inter-PCT investigation team ...	5.31	Agree.
15b	...or, in a case raising difficult or complex issues, by the Healthcare Commission. Consideration should be given to amending the relevant provisions of the draft Complaints Regulations to permit the Healthcare Commission to accept and investigate concerns referred to it by a PCT or healthcare body without the need for a reference from the Secretary of State for Health.		See above on recommendation 13.
16	Objective standards, by reference to which complaints can be judged, should be established as a matter of urgency. These standards should be applied by those making the decision whether to uphold or reject a complaint and by PCTs and other NHS bodies when deciding what actions to take in respect of a doctor against whom a complaint has been upheld. When established, the standards by reference to which complaints are dealt with must fit together with the threshold by reference to which the GMC will accept and act upon allegations, so as to form a comprehensive framework.	5.16	Agree; a study led by CHRE is developing protocols for local investigations, including defining the thresholds at which cases should be referred to the professional regulator.
17	In order to ensure that, so far as possible, complaints about healthcare can reach the appropriate destinations, there should be a 'single portal' by which complaints or concerns can be directed or redirected to the appropriate quarter. This service should also provide information about the various advice services available to persons who are considering whether and/or how to complain or raise a concern. Advice must be provided for persons who are concerned about the legal implications of raising a concern.		Accept need for better support for patients who are unsure where to make a complaint. Preferred solution is to introduce standards so that all bodies receiving complaints will forward to right recipient and tell complainant what they have done.
18	About two years after the Complaints regulations come into force in their entirety, and independent review should be commissioned into the operation of the new arrangements for advising and supporting patients who wish to make a complaint.		Agree in principle and will link with the planned review of the NHS redress scheme (three years after implementation).

Rec	Inquiry recommendation	Government response	
		Para	**Response**
19	The powers of PCTs should be extended so as to enable them to issue warnings to GPs and to impose financial penalties on GPs in respect of misconduct, deficient professional performance or deficient clinical practice which falls below the thresholds for referral to the GMC or exercise of the PCT's list management powers.		Agree in principle and will discuss with stakeholders as part of the broader review of the Performers List system.
20	Steps should be taken to ensure that every prescription generated by a GP can be accurately attributed to an individual doctor. Only then will the data resulting from the monitoring of prescribing information constitute a reliable clinical governance tool.	8.10	Work is already in hand to implement this recommendation, based on the linked recommendation in the Inquiry's Fourth Report. The intention is that every prescriber will be identified by a unique 12-digit number which, for GPs, would incorporate the GP's unique GMC reference number while indicating the PCT and the GP practice.
21	Regular monitoring of GPs' prescribing should be undertaken by PCTs. Special attention should be paid to the prescribing of controlled drugs by GPs. Doctors who have had a problem of drug misuse in the past or who are suspected of having a current problem should be subjected to particularly close scrutiny.	8.10	PCTs already routinely monitor prescribing by GPs and other prescribers. The government will invite the RCGP to work with the NHS Information Centre on how such information can best be used to assure the quality of GP services.
21	When a restriction is placed on a doctor's prescribing powers, this information must be made available (preferably by electronic means) to those who need to know, particularly pharmacists.		Accepted – see the government response to the Inquiry's 4th report, recommendation 8. For doctors, the GMC's web based database of doctor's registration already contains details of any restrictions on a doctor's practice.
22	The Department of Health (DoH) should make provision for a national system for monitoring GP patient mortality rates. The system should be supported by a well organised, consistent and objective means of investigating those cases where a GP's patient mortality rates signal as being above the norm.	8.12	The NHS Information Centre has developed and rolled out a Primary Care Mortality Database. We will evaluate after 12 months the extent to which this has provided useful information to PCTs. Early experience suggests that practice-level mortality data, on its own, may only have limited use for clinical governance purposes.
23	Every GP practice should keep a death register in which the particulars of the deaths of patients of the practice should be recorded for use in audit and for other purposes.	8.13	Accept and will be take forward with GP representatives as part of the consultation on death certification.

Rec	Inquiry recommendation	Government response	
		Para	Response
24	PCTs should undertake reviews of the medical records of deceased patients, either on a routine periodic basis (if resources permit) or on a targeted basis limited to those GPs whose performance gives rise to concern.		As for previous recommendation.
25	The purpose of GP appraisal must be made clear. A decision must be taken as to whether it is intended to be a purely formative (i.e. educational) process or whether it is intended to serve several purposes: part formative, part summative (i.e. pass/fail) and/or part performance management.		Accept. Appraisal for doctors will in future have a summative component and will be an integral part of the government's proposals for revalidation. *See Trust, assurance and safety* chapter 2.
26	If appraisal is intended to be a clinical governance tool, it must be 'toughened up'. If that is to be done, the following steps will be necessary. Appraiser should be more thoroughly trained and accredited following some form of test or assessment. Appraisers should be trained to evaluate the appraisee's fitness to practise. GPs should be appraised by GPs from another PCT. Standards must be specified, by which a GP 'successfully completes' or 'fails' the appraisal. All appraisals should be based on a nationally agreed core of verifiable information supplied by the PCT to both the appraiser and the appraisee.		As for previous recommendation.
27	The Family Health Services Authority (Special Health Authority) or its proposed successor, the NHS litigation Authority, should collect and analyse information relating to the use made by PCTs of their list management powers. Such analysis would assist the DoH in providing guidance to PCTs about the types of circumstance in which they might properly use their powers.	4.37–38	FHSAA already publish some relevant analyses. In light of the findings of a report commissioned by DH from the Sheffield School of Health and Allied Research, we feel it would be unreasonable to ask PCTs to report further data.
28	The Government should consider the feasibility of providing a financial incentive for the achievement of GP practice accreditation by means of a scheme similar to that operated by the Royal College of General Practitioners in Scotland.	4.39	The Royal College of General Practitioners has been developing proposals for a Primary Care Practice Accreditation Scheme, based on its current Quality Team Development scheme. The government is considering as part of its wider programme of system reform.

Rec	Inquiry recommendation	Government response	
		Para	Response
29	The policy of the DoH and PCTs should be to focus on the resolution of the problems inherent in single-handed and small practices. More support and encouragement should be given to GPs running single-handed and small practices. In return, more should be expected of such GPs in terms of group activity and mutual supervision. Initiatives such as the sharing of staff, mentoring and peer support schemes that promote the 'cross-fertilisation' of staff between one single-handed or small GP practice and another should be encouraged wherever possible. The DoH should take responsibility for these initiatives.	4.42	Agree in principle and will discuss with new PCTs and other interested parties how to take forward.
30	PCTs should be willing and able to provide advice to GP practices on good recruitment practice and should also be willing to offer support in drafting job specifications and advertisements. They should be prepared, if requested, to assist in sifting applications (if multiple applications are received) and in making the necessary checks on applications before the interview stage, so as to exclude in advance any applicants who are unsuitable. However, this latter exercise may be too much of a burden for PCTs unless and until the Inquiry's recommendations for greater information to be placed on the GMC's website and for the creation of a central database of information about doctors (see below) are implemented.	4.40	As for previous recommendation.
31	A standard reference form should be developed for use in connection with appointments to GP practices. PCTs should insist that a reference is obtained from the doctor's previous employer or PCT. In the case of a PCT, the reference should be signed by the Medical Director or Clinical Governance Lead.	4.40	As for previous recommendation.
32	When recruiting a new member, GP practices should canvass and take account of the views of their patients about the kind of doctor the practice needs.	4.40	Agree that practices should be responsive to the views of their patients in deciding how to develop their services. Ultimately however practices must remain accountable for the way in which those services are provided, including any new appointments.

Rec	Inquiry recommendation	Government response	
		Para	Response
33	PCTs should keep a separate file for each individual GP on their lists. That file should hold all material relating to the doctor which could have any possible relevance to clinical governance. If a doctor moves from one PCT to another, the file (or a copy of it) should be sent to the new PCT.	8.3	Accept in principle, and will take forward in discussion with stakeholders.
33	It might be helpful if the DoH were to establish national criteria for the content of the files to be kept by PCTs.	8.6	Accept.
34a	Every GP practice should have a written policy, setting out the procedure to be followed by a member of the practice staff who wishes to raise concerns, in particular concerns about the clinical practice or conduct of a healthcare professional within the practice. Staff should be encouraged to bring forward any concerns they may have openly, routinely and without fear of criticism.	5.33	All NHS organisations should have such a policy; will discuss with stakeholders how best to carry forward.
34b	In the event that a member of the staff of a GP practice feels unable to raise his/her concern within the practice, s/he should be able to approach a person designated by the PCT for the purpose. The contact details of that person should appear in the written policy. The designated person should make him/herself known to all practice staff working in the PCT area. PCTs should ensure, through training, that practice staff understand the importance of reporting concerns and know how to do so.	5.35	Accept in principle that an appropriate channel for such concerns should be available. Either the PCT or SHA may have a role; will discuss further with stakeholders.
35	The written policy should contain details of organisations from which staff can obtain free independent advice. If the 'single portal' is created, in whatever form, the policy should set out contact details of that also.	5.33	Accept.
36	It should be a statutory requirement for all private healthcare organisations to have a clear written policy for the raising of concerns. Steps should be taken to foster in the private sector the same culture of openness that is being encouraged in the NHS.	5.36	Agree in principle but will secure through the new regulatory arrangements which will apply to all healthcare providers.
37	Consideration should be given to amending the Public Interest Disclosure Act 1998 in order to give greater protection to persons disclosing information, the disclosure of which is in the public interest.	5.38	Not persuaded that change to PIDA is needed. Will work with NHS organisations to draw up protocols under Act which will give equivalent protection to that sought by Inquiry.

Rec	Inquiry recommendation	Government response	
		Para	Response
38	Written policies setting out procedures for raising concerns in the healthcare sector should be capable of being used in relation to persons who do not share a common employment.	5.39	Accept.
39	There should be some national provision (probably a telephone helpline) to enable any person, whether working within heath care or not, to obtain advice about the best way to raise a concern about a healthcare matter and about the legal implications of doing so. It might be possible to link this helpline with the 'single portal' previously referred to.		We will discuss with SHAs and PCTs the best way of providing a locally or regionally based helpline for health service staff, or members of the general public, who want confidential advice about raising concerns. This could be linked to the service described in the response to recommendation 34.
40	There should be a central database containing information about every doctor working in the UK. This should be accessible to the officers of NHS bodies and to accredited employers in the private sector, as well as to other bodies with a legitimate interest, such as the Healthcare Commission, the GMC, the NCAA [NCAS]and the DoH.	8.7	Accept in principle; the Department will discuss with stakeholders how the GMC register could be enhanced to provide this resource (see *Trust, assurance and safety* chapter 6).
41	The database would contain, or provide links to, information held by the GMC, the Criminal Records Bureau (CRB) and the NHS Counter Fraud and Security Management Service. It would also contain records of disciplinary action by employers, details of list management action by PCTs, any adverse reports following the investigation of a complaint, any adverse findings by a Healthcare Commission panel or by the Healthcare Ombudsman and details of any findings of negligence in a clinical negligence action and settlement of a clinical negligence claim above a pre-determined level of damages. It should also contain certain other information. Doctors would be able to access their own entries to check the accuracy of the information held.	8.7	As for previous recommendation.
42	Private sector employers should be required to provide relevant information as a condition of registration with the Healthcare Commission.	8.7	As for previous recommendation.
42	Deputising services should also be required to provide information and should be able to access the database through the relevant PCT.	8.7	As for previous recommendation.

Rec	Inquiry recommendation	Government response	
		Para	Response
43	Information about unsubstantiated allegations or concerns should not be included on the central database. Instead, the doctor's entry on the database should be flagged to indicate that confidential information is held by a named NHS body or by the CRB or the GMC or the NHS Counter Fraud and Security Management Service. Questions of access to that information would depend on who was asking for it and for what purpose and would have to be determined at a high level.	8.7	As for previous recommendation.
44	GPs should be required to disclose to the relevant PCT the fact that a clinical negligence claim has been brought against them, the gist of the allegation made and, when the time comes, the outcome of the claim.	8.14	The government is sympathetic to the intention behind this recommendation but recognises that it raises some practical issues. Will discuss further with stakeholders.
45	The GMC should adopt a policy of tiered disclosure to apply to all persons seeking information about a doctor.	8.15	We understand that the GMC has already introduced a system of tiered disclosure after consultation with stakeholders.
46	The first tier should relate to information which is relevant to the doctor's current registration status, together with certain information about his/her past fitness to practise (FTP) history. First tier information should be posted on the GMC website and should also be disclosed to anyone who requests information about the doctor's registration. The periods of time for which information should remain at the first tier should depend on the nature of the information. When the relevant period expires, the information should be removed from the website. It should be replaced by a note indicating that there is further information which can be obtained by telephoning the GMC. That information should then be available at the second tier.	8.15	As for previous recommendation.
47	Disclosure of information at the second tier should be made to any person who makes a request about a doctor's FTP history. All information which has at any time been in the public domain should remain available to enquirers at the second tier for as long as the doctor remains on the register.	8.15	As for previous recommendation.

Rec	Inquiry recommendation	Government response	
		Para	Response
48	In all cases where a GP's registration is subject to conditions, or where s/he has resumed practice after a period of suspension or erasure, patients of any practice in which the GP works should be told. A letter of explanation which has been approved by the PCT, should be sent to all patients. Patients should have the opportunity to refuse to be treated by a doctor who is subject to conditions or who has previously been subject to an order for suspension or erasure.	8.16	Accept in principle but need to strike careful balance between informing patients and helping the rehabilitation of the individual doctor. Will discuss further with NHS, professional and patient groups.
49	The GMC should ensure that its publications contain accurate and readily understandable guidance as to the types of case that do and do not fall within the remit of its FTP procedures.		The GMC accepts this recommendation. In particular: 1. The GMC has revised and published a new leaflet for patients. The leaflet includes examples of the types of case that the GMC will investigate. 2. All of the GMC's decision-making guidance is publicly available, including examples of the types of cases where failure to meet standards may lead to action on registration. 3. The GMC re-launched its core guidance to doctors, *Good Medical Practice*, in November 2006. The online versions provides links to examples of cases heard by GMC panels where a failure to follow the guidance led to action by the GMC.
50	There must be complete separation of the GMC's casework and governance functions at the investigation stage of the new FTP procedures and this must be reflected in the Rules.		The GMC accepts this principle and the required separation was introduced in November 2004.
51	The adjudication stage of the FTP procedures must be undertaken by a body independent of the GMC. This body should appoint and train lay and medically qualified panellists and take on the task of appointing case managers, legal assessors (if they are still necessary) and any necessary specialist advisors. It should also provide administrative support for hearings.		Accept – see *Trust, assurance and safety* Chapter 4

Rec	Inquiry recommendation	Government response	
		Para	**Response**
52	Consideration should be given to appointing a body of full-time, or nearly full-time, panellists who could sit on the FTP panels of all the healthcare regulatory bodies.		Accept – see *Trust, assurance and safety* Chapter 4
53	The GMC should adopt clear, objective tests to be applied by decision-makers at the investigation and adjudication stages of the FTP procedures. The tests that I recommend are set out at paragraphs 25.63 and 25.67–25.68. The tests should be incorporated in the Medical Act 1983 and/or in the Rules. The draft Guidance for panellists should be amended so that it is consistent with the provisions of section 35D of the Medical Act 1983 and rule 17(2)(k) of the November 2004 Rules.		The GMC has amended its draft guidance for panellists to ensure that it is consistent with the provisions of Section 35D of the Medical Act 1983 and rule 17(2)(k) of the General Medical Council (Fitness to Practise) Rules Order 2004. The Department of Health intends to commission a review of the GMC's processes four years after the introduction of the reformed procedures (see recommendation 105). The tests applied at the investigation and adjudication stages will be reviewed at that point and this will include a discussion with key stakeholders to ensure that tests are consistent across all regulatory bodies.
54	The Medical Act 1983 should be amended to add a further route by which there might be a finding of impairment of fitness to practise, namely 'deficient clinical practise'.		The Government is not persuaded that there is a need for this further category.
55	Urgent steps should be taken to develop standards, criteria and thresholds so that decision-makers will be able to reach reasonably consistent decisions at both the investigation and the adjudication stages of the FTP procedures and on restoration applications.		The GMC has developed detailed guidance for its decision-makers at the investigation and adjudication stages of the FTP procedures. As noted above, this guidance includes examples of the types of cases where failure to meet standards may put registration at risk. In addition, as noted above, the online version of the November 2006 update of *Good Medical Practice* provides links to examples of cases heard by GMC panels where a failure to follow the guidance led to action on registration.

Rec	Inquiry recommendation	Government response	
		Para	Response
56	The Council for the Regulation of Healthcare Professionals (now known as the Council for Healthcare Regulatory Excellence (CRHP/CHRE)) should be invited to set up a panel of professional and lay people (similar in nature to the Sentencing Advisory Panel) which should assist in the process of developing the necessary standards, criteria and thresholds.		The Government agrees that the CHRE can play a valuable role in promoting greater consistency in standards between the professional regulators. This is likely to be an increasingly important aspect of its work – see *Trust, assurance and safety* para 1.25.
57	Steps should be taken to ensure that FTP panels determining cases in which issues of deficient professional performance arise apply a standard which is no lower than that set for admission to general practice.		The Government agrees with the GMC's view that individuals should be assessed on the basis of their particular experience and expertise. The GMC is working on assessment tools in each specialty that reflect this approach.
58	Rule 4 of the General Medical Council (Fitness to Practise) Rules Order of Council 2004 (the November 2004 Rules), which sets out the test to be applied by the Registrar on receipt of an allegation, should be amended to give greater clarity. The recommended test is set out at paragraph 25.125.		The GMC have clarified the test to be applied by the Registrar and have redrafted the guidance to the FTP rules to reflect this clarification. The GMC has made a number of other changes to the guidance to the rules and will shortly be consulting on the revised guidance.
59	The November 2004 Rules should be amended to make formal provision for the GMC routinely to communicate with employers and with primary care organisations (PCOs) before deciding what action should be taken in response to an allegation and giving the GMC power to require from the doctor the necessary details to enable it to make such communication. Communication should take place in all cases other than in the case of an allegation which is so serious that it obviously requires further investigation or an allegation which is plainly outside the GMC's remit.	See paras 4.20–24	The Government agrees that the GMC should routinely involve employers and PCTs in deciding how cases should be handled; this is now standard practice following the 2004 changes to the FTP procedures. In future, many more cases will be handled locally in discussion between the local employer or PCT and the GMC affiliate.

Rec	Inquiry recommendation	Government response	
		Para	**Response**
60	Where a doctor has committed a criminal offence in respect of which a court has imposed a conditional discharge, that offence should be dealt with by the GMC in the same way as if it were a criminal conviction.		The Fitness to Practise rules provide that all convictions resulting in a custodial sentences must be referred by the Registrar directly to a FTP panel. The Registrar has a discretion to refer for all other convictions and cautions. At the adjudication stage, a certificate of conviction is conclusive evidence of the offence committed. The Department of Health intends to commission a review of the GMC's processes four years after the introduction of the reformed procedures (see recommendation 105). The treatment of conditional discharges will be considered at that point.
61	The November 2004 Rules should be amended so as to give case examiners, and Investigation Committee (IC) panels in cases where the case examiners have disagreed, the power to direct investigations.		Case examiners and the Investigation Committee can seek any information or evidence they need before making a decision on a case. The guidance to the FTP rules has been redrafted to reflect this. The GMC intends to consult on the revised guidance shortly.
62	Case examiners should be advised that they should not take mitigation into account when making their decisions and that they should consult a lawyer if they are in any doubt as to whether the available evidence is such that there is a realistic prospect of proving the allegation.		Case examiners are advised to consult a lawyer where there are any concerns about the available evidence. The GMC now has in-house lawyers to support investigations and provide advice to decision-makers at the investigation stage of the FTP. The GMC has advised case examiners not to take mitigation into account when making decisions.

Rec	Inquiry recommendation	Government response	
		Para	**Response**
63	The November 2004 Rules should be amended to give case examiners, and Investigation Committee (IC) panels in cases where the case examiners have disagreed, the power to direct that an assessment of a doctor's performance and/or health should be carried out.		Case examiners and the Investigation Committee can seek any information or evidence they need before making a decision on a case, which would include an assessment of a doctor's performance or health. This is reflected in the guidance on the investigation stage test which is available on the GMC website. The guidance to the FTP rules has been redrafted to reflect this. The GMC intends to consult on the revised guidance shortly.
64	The GMC should develop an abridged performance assessment to be used as a screening tool in any case in which an allegation is made which potentially calls into question the quality of a doctor's clinical practice.		The GMC has undertaken extensive work with the Royal Colleges on the development of assessment instruments for modular assessment and is intending to pilot the approach in general practice in 2007. Some changes to the FTP Rules 2004 may be required before the GMC could apply a modular or abridged approach to performance assessment.
65	In order to avoid doctors undergoing multiple performance assessments, the GMC should investigate the development of a modular assessment.		See previous recommendation.
66	The November 2004 Rules should be amended to include a provision whereby reports of performance assessments should be disclosed by the GMC to doctors' employers or PCOs as soon as possible after receipt.		The duty to share the performance assessment report with an employer is in the rules at Rule 7(5) of the General Medical Council (Fitness to Practise) Rules 2004.
67	The power to send letters of advice should be incorporated into the Rules and clear criteria for the sending of such letters should be prepared.		The power to send letters of advice is now incorporated in the revised guidance to the FTP rules on which the GMC will shortly be consulting. The guidance includes reference to the types of case in which a letter of advice may be the appropriate response. In future many more cases may, subject to the outcome of piloting, be handled locally in discussion between the local employer or PCT and the GMC affiliate.

Rec	Inquiry recommendation	Government response	
		Para	Response
68	The GMC should reconsider its proposals for the issuing of warnings at the investigation stage.		The GMC has been closely monitoring the issuing of warnings at the investigation stage and is satisfied that this is working effectively. In future, many cases of this kind are likely to be handled at local level through issuing Recorded Concerns or agreeing remedial packages.
69	Rule 28 of the November 2004 Rules, which provides for the cancellation of hearings before a FTP panel, should be amended so as to provide that a decision to cancel must be taken by an Investigation Committee panel and that the reasons for the cancellation must be formally recorded. Both the doctor and maker of the allegation should be notified in advance of the fact that cancellation is being considered and both should have the opportunity to make representations.		The GMC have redrafted the guidance to the FTP rules and will shortly be consulting on this draft. The guidance now provides that representations will be sought from the practitioner and the maker of the allegation. There is separate draft guidance for decision-makers on dealing with applications for cancellations. The Department of Health intends to commission a review of the GMC's processes four years after the introduction of the reformed procedures (see recommendation 105). The process for considering applications for cancellation will be reviewed at that point.
70	There should be regular monitoring and audit of the number of applications to cancel FTP panel hearings and of the decisions to cancel and the reasons for those applications and decisions. Those reasons should be scrutinised with a view to taking steps to minimise the number of cases in which referrals are subsequently cancelled. The number and reasons should be placed in the public domain on an annual basis.		The GMC undertakes quality assurance of decisions to cancel referrals and is reviewing the information published on its FTP procedures. The introduction of a new IT system in 2006 will enable the GMC to publish fuller and more detailed statistical information. The Department looks forward to seeing the GMC's proposals, in particular how the GMC proposes to discharge its new direct accountability to Parliament.

Rec	Inquiry recommendation	Government response	
		Para	Response
71	If the GMC pursues its present intention to extend the use of voluntary undertakings to cases other than those raising issues of adverse health or deficient performance, the disposal of such cases should take place in public at the adjudication stage and not in private as part of the investigation stage.		Provision for consensual disposal was included in the Medical Act and Miscellaneous Amendments Order 2006. The GMC will consult on amended rules in 2007. Undertakings restricting a doctor's practice will be published on the GMC Register and monitored in the same way as conditions imposed by a panel; and workplace and medical supervisors will be appointed to support the remediation and re-training process. In future many cases of this kind may, subject to the outcome of piloting, be handled through the Recorded Concern procedure and voluntary agreements monitored by local employers in consultation with the GMC affiliate.
72	The November 2004 Rules should be amended to make provision for the revival of closed allegations. The usual 'cut-off' period should be five years but it should be possible, in exceptional circumstances and in the interests of patient protection, to reopen a case at any time.		In the light of cases such as those of Shipman and Ayling the Department agrees that "closed" allegations could in certain circumstances have continuing relevance to the protection of patients, eg in combination with newer information. There are however complex legal and ethical issues; the GMC has received legal advice that an unfettered discretion to re-open a case at any time could be open to legal challenge. The Department will discuss the options further with the GMC as part of discussion of the content of local files (see recommendation 33 above) and the introduction of Recorded Concerns.
73	Reviews of investigation stage decisions should be carried out by an independent external commissioner. The circumstances in which a review may take place should be extended to cover decisions of the Registrar to reject an allegation rather than to refer it to a case examiner.		The Department agrees that a sample of decisions at the investigation stage should be subject to independent audit by CHRE; see *Trust, assurance and safety* para 4.16.

Rec	Inquiry recommendation	Government response	
		Para	Response
74	The November 2004 Rules should be amended so as to provide that the arrangements for the obtaining and consideration of health assessments and for the management and supervision of doctors who are the subject of voluntary undertakings relating to health should be directed by a medically qualified case examiner, who should fulfil the functions previously carried out by a health screener. If a case is to be closed on the basis of a health assessment, the decision should be taken by two case examiners, one medically qualified and one lay and, if they disagree, by an IC panel.		Agreed – this reflects existing practice and policy and is covered in GMC guidance. The rules state that all decisions to close a case at the end of an investigation must be taken by two case examiners, one medical and one lay. The GMC has redrafted its guidance to the FTP rules to reflect current practice and intends to consult on this guidance shortly.
75	The November 2004 Rules should be amended so as to provide that the arrangements for the obtaining and consideration of performance assessments and for the management and supervision of doctors who are the subject of voluntary undertakings relating to performance should be directed by a medically qualified case examiner, who should fulfil the functions previously carried out by a performance case co-ordinator. If a case is to be closed on the basis of a performance assessment, the decision should be taken by two case examiners, one medically qualified and one lay and, if they disagree, by an IC panel.		As for previous recommendation.
76	There should be an explicit power in the Rules to allow the GMC to undertake any further investigations it considers necessary after a case has been referred to a FTP panel and before the panel hearing.		This reflects existing GMC policy and practice. The GMC has redrafted its guidance to the FTP rules to reflect current practice and intends to consult on this guidance shortly.
77	In the event that the GMC retains control of the adjudication stage, the GMC committee charged with governance of the adjudication stage should audit the work of case managers. Case management should apply to cases with a performance element.		This recommendation will be brought to the attention of the independent adjudicator in due course. In the meanwhile, the GMC has ensured that case management applies in all places, and has in place a process in place to review and quality assure decisions taken by its case managers. The GMC has redrafted its guidance to the FTP rules to reflect this practice.

Rec	Inquiry recommendation	Government response	
		Para	**Response**
78	FTP panellists should be warned that they should exercise caution about drawing adverse inferences from a failure to comply with case management orders.		We will draw this recommendation to the attention of the independent adjudicator in due course. In the meanwhile the GMC has revised its guidance to reflect this point.
79	In the event that the GMC retains control of the adjudication stage, it should appoint a number of legally qualified chairmen who should, as an experiment or pilot, preside over the more complex FTP panel hearings. The results of the pilot scheme should be scrutinised to see whether there are benefits, whether in terms of the improved conduct of hearings, more consistent outcomes, improved reasons and/or fewer appeals.		We will draw this recommendation to the attention of the independent adjudicator.
80	As part of their training, FTP panellists should be advised about their discretion to admit hearsay evidence and other forms of evidence not admissible in a criminal trial. Panellists should also be advised, during training, that it is entirely appropriate for them to intervene during FTP panel hearings and to ask questions if they feel that any issue is not being adequately explored.		This is now included in GMC guidance and training for panellists.
81	The GMC should reopen its debate about the standard of proof to be applied by FTP panels. It should consider introducing a rule that the civil standard of proof should apply unless the doctor faces an allegation of misconduct which also amounts to a serious criminal offence. In that limited class of case, the criminal standard of proof may well be appropriate.		The Government has decided that all health professions regulators should follow the civil standard of proof. It should be flexibly applied to take into account the circumstances and gravity of individual cases.
82	The GMC should abandon its intention to notify doctors, at the same time as sending notice of referral of their case to a FTP panel, of the outcome it will be seeking at the FTP panel hearing.		The GMC have revised their guidance and no longer adopt this approach.
83	FTP panels should be required to give brief reasons for their main findings of fact.		As for recommendation 79.
84	Rule 17(5)(b) of the November 2004 Rules (which permits a FTP panel, on receipt of a report of a health or performance assessment, to refer the allegation back into the investigation stage for consideration of voluntary undertakings) should be revoked.		As for recommendation 79. Although only the most potentially serious cases will need to go to the independent adjudicator, the government believes that, even at this stage, remedial action based on voluntary undertakings should remain one option.

Rec	Inquiry recommendation	Government response	
		Para	**Response**
85	Rule 17(2)(j) of the November 2004 Rules should be amended to make clear what types of further evidence should be received before a FTP panel decides whether a doctor's fitness to practise is impaired. That evidence should include the doctor's previous FTP history with the GMC or any other regulatory body. Rule 17(2)(l) should be amended to make clear what categories of evidence might be received after a finding of impairment of fitness to practise but before determination of sanction.		This reflects existing GMC policy and practice. The GMC has redrafted its guidance to the FTP rules to reflect this practice and intends to consult on this guidance shortly. The recommendation will be brought to the attention of the independent adjudicator in due course.
86	The Medical Act 1983 should be amended to permit a FTP panel to issue a warning in a case where it has found that a doctor's fitness to practice is impaired but not to a degree justifying action on registration.		The Department will in due course seek the views of the independent adjudicator and other stakeholders on this recommendation.
87	Rule 17(2)(m) of the November 2004 Rules, which permits a FTP panel to take into account written undertakings entered into by a doctor when deciding how to deal with the doctor's case, should be revoked. If it is to be retained, the rule should be amended to make clear that undertakings can be taken into account only at the stage of deciding on sanction, after findings of fact and a decision about impairment to practise have been made. In that event also, provision should be made within the Rules for supervision of the doctor to ensure compliance with undertakings, for the holding of review hearings in cases where a doctor has given undertakings and for dealing with a breach of an undertaking.		This reflects current GMC policy and practice, and guidance to the FTP rules has been redrafted to reflect this. The recommendation will be brought to the attention of the independent adjudicator in due course.
88	Throughout the period that a doctor's registration is subject to conditions imposed by a FTP panel or to voluntary undertakings, someone within the GMC (preferably a case examiner) should take responsibility for the doctor's progress and for ensuring, so far as possible, that s/he is complying with the conditions imposed or undertakings given.		Agreed. This reflects current policy and practice. The GMC established a Case Review team in 2004 to undertake this work. The GMC appoints medical supervisors and workplace supervisors as appropriate and members of the Case Review team liaise with these supervisors to ensure that the doctor is complying with any conditions or undertakings. Medically qualified case examiners are involved in the review process. These arrangements will be reviewed once the independent adjudicator has been set up.

Rec	Inquiry recommendation	Government response	
		Para	**Response**
89	In every case where a doctor is continuing to practise subject to conditions or voluntary undertakings, a professional supervisor should be appointed to oversee and report on the doctor's progress and on his/her compliance with the conditions or undertakings. In a case where a doctor's health is an issue, a medical supervisor should be appointed.		See previous recommendation.
90	Any breach of a condition imposed by a FTP panel or of a voluntary undertaking (save for the most minor breach) should result in the doctor being referred back (or referred) to a FTP panel so that consideration can be given to imposing a sanction which affords a greater degree of protection to the public.		Agreed in principle – this reflects current GMC policy as set out in the revised guidance to the FTP rules. Further discussion will be needed on how to put this principle into effect once the independent adjudicator has been set up.
91	The November 2005 Rules should be amended to ensure that there is at least one review hearing in all cases where a period of suspension or conditions on registration have been imposed, unless there are exceptional reasons why no such hearing should take place.		This reflects current GMC policy and practice and guidance to the FTP rules has been redrafted to reflect this. The recommendation will be brought to the attention of the independent adjudicator in due course.
92	The arrangements set out in the 2003 draft Rules, whereby any necessary gathering of evidence in preparation for a review hearing would be undertaken by a specially appointed case examiner, should be reinstated.		Under current GMC policy , case examiners are involved in preparing cases for review where the conditions relate to a doctor's performance or health. The GMC have redrafted guidance to the FTP rules to reflect this and will be consulting on that guidance shortly.
93	In all but exceptional cases, a doctor whose registration has been suspended should be required to undergo an objective assessment of his/her fitness to practise before being permitted to return to practice. That assessment should be considered by a FTP panel at a review hearing and a decision should be taken as to the doctor's fitness to practise. A doctor who has been the subject of conditions on his/her registration should be required to go through the same process. Doctors who are the subject of voluntary undertakings should also be required to undergo an appropriate assessment before their undertakings are permitted to lapse.		The Government agrees in principle with this recommendation, although in certain circumstances the evidence gathered for revalidation may be sufficient to establish objective evidence of fitness to practice. Existing GMC rules give the Registrar the power to require the doctor to undergo an assessment but that power is discretionary. We suggest that the GMC should discuss the recommendation further with the independent adjudicator when established.

Rec	Inquiry recommendation	Government response	
		Para	Response
94	The GMC's primary role should be one, not of remediation of doctors, but of protection of patients. If a doctor who is subject to conditions or voluntary undertakings undergoes an assessment in the circumstances described above, and the assessment reveals that s/he does not meet the required standard, consideration should be given to taking the steps necessary to remove the doctor from practice. He or she should not be permitted to 'limp on' with repeated periods of conditional registration and no real hope of meeting the standard for unrestricted practice.		The Government agrees with that the primary role of regulation should be to protect patients. This principle underlies the proposals in *Trust, assurance and safety* on revalidation, remediation and rehabilitation. It is also reflected in the GMC's current Indicative Sanctions Guidance for FTP panellists. At present, erasure is not available for those doctors whose fitness to practise is impaired solely by reason of ill-health, but indefinite suspension is available. Further discussion will be needed once the independent adjudicator is established.
95	The arrangements set out in the 2003 draft Rules, whereby any necessary gathering of evidence in preparation for a restoration hearing should be undertaken by a specially appointed case examiner, should be reinstated.		Current GMC policy is that, on receipt of an application for restoration, the Registrar may make any investigation he considers appropriate including requiring the applicant to undergo a performance or health assessment. Case examiners will be involved where a performance or health assessment is undertaken. We suggest that the GMC should discuss the recommendation further with the independent adjudicator when established.
96	Every doctor whose application for restoration to the register has reached the second stage of the procedure should be required to undergo an objective assessment of every aspect of his/her fitness to practise. The doctor should not be restored to the register unless s/he has met the required standard.		The Government agrees in principle with this recommendation. Existing rules give the Registrar the power to require the applicant to undergo an assessment but that power is discretionary. In practice, FTP panels often require an assessment at this stage of the process.

Rec	Inquiry recommendation	Government response	
		Para	**Response**
97	Doctors who are restored to the register should be required to have a mentor whose task it will be to monitor, and report to the GMC on, their progress in practice.		Agreed. *Trust, assurance and safety* addresses the need for employers to work closely with the GMC affiliate to ensure that doctors who are continuing to work under conditions, or who are restored to the register following erasure, are given the help and support they need.
98	A thorough investigation of the circumstances underlying allegations of misconduct involving drug abuse should be conducted. The full facts should be established, including the circumstances in which the abuse began.		Agreed – the GMC's reformed fitness to practise procedures allow for this as it can now investigate both the conduct issues and any underlying health problem and review the doctor's fitness to practise in the round. The national advisory group, which will be advising on a national strategy to ensure the health of health professionals, will be asked in particular to consider the need for access to addiction services (see *Trust, assurance and safety* paras 4.28–30).
99	The GMC should commission research into drug abusing doctors and their outcomes following supervision under the health procedures.		Agreed – we will discuss further with the GMC who have entered into a strategic partnership with the Economic and Social Research Council to fund a research programme on medical regulation. One of the areas to be explored is risk factors in professional performance.
100	Every aspect of the FTP procedures in which either doctors or makers of allegations have direct interest should be set out in the Rules		Reject. The Department's policy is that general powers and principles should be included in the relevant Order, while matters concerning the rights and duties of individuals and organisations should be in Rules, with operational detail set out transparently in published guidance.

Rec	Inquiry recommendation	Government response	
		Para	Response
100	In addition, the GMC should publish a FTP manual, containing all its relevant Rules and its guidance for panellists, case examiners and staff, together with any relevant Standing Orders.		Agreed. All of the GMC's rules and decision-making guidance, including examples of the types of cases where failure to meet standards may lead to action on registration, is now published on the GMC's website. We will in due course draw this attention to the independent adjudicator to ensure that guidance on all stages of the FTP processes will continue to be publicly available.
101	Clear statistical information should be collected and published by the GMC. The GMC should publish an annual report which should amount to a transparent statement of the year's activities in respect of the FTP procedures.		Agreed. The GMC has recently introduced a new IT system which will allow them to gather and publish much more detailed information about the FTP procedures. The Department looks forward to seeing the GMC's proposals for the information to be published.
102	The GMC should carry out audits of various aspects of its procedures, in addition to its other routine auditing activities.		Agreed. All aspects of the GMC's procedures as well as decisions at the investigation stage of the process and at the adjudication stage of the process are subject to regular review and quality assurance. A full audit programme of GMC procedures takes place under the auspices of the Audit Committee. In addition, as described above under recommendation 73, the Government will invite CHRE to audit a sample of decisions from the GMC's FTP processes.
103	The arrangements for revalidation should be amended so that revalidation comprises, as required by section 29A of the Medical Act 1983, an evaluation of an individual doctor's fitness to practise.		Agreed – see *Trust, assurance and safety* chapter 2.
104	The annual report referred to at 101 above should include clear statistical information about the number of applications for revalidation and their outcomes. It should amount to a transparent statement of the year's revalidation activities.		The GMC agrees in principle with this recommendation and will review its plans in the light of the approach to revalidation set out in *Trust, assurance and safety*.

Rec	Inquiry recommendation	Government response	
		Para	Response
105	In three to four year's time, there should be a thorough review of the operation of the new FTP procedures, to be carried out by an independent organisation. This task should be undertaken by or on the instructions of the CRHP/CHRE.		Agreed – the Department proposes to commission a review of the GMC's new FTP processes 4 years after their introduction, ie during 2009. We agree that this would be an appropriate task for CHRE and will discuss this suggestion with them in due course.
106	The GMC's constitution should be reconsidered, with view to changing its balance, so that elected medical members do not have an overall majority. Medical and lay members who are to be appointed (by the Privy Council) should be selected for nomination to the Privy Council by the Public Appointments Commission following open competition.		Agreed – see *Trust, assurance and safety* chapter 1.
107	The GMC should be directly accountable to Parliament and should publish an annual report which should be scrutinised by a Parliamentary Select Committee.		Agreed – see *Trust, assurance and safety* chapter 1.
108	Section 29 of the National Health Service Reform and Health Care Professions Act 2002 should be amended so as to clarify that the Act provides for the CRHP/CHRE to appeal against 'acquittals' and findings of no impairment of fitness to practise, as well as in respect of sanctions which it believes were unduly lenient.		The Government understands that a recent case in the Court of Appeal has already established this principle.
109	There should in the future be a review of the powers of the CRHP/CHRE with a view to ascertaining whether any extension of its powers and functions is necessary in order to enable it to act effectively to ensure that patients are sufficiently protected by the GMC.		Chapter 1 of *Trust, assurance and safety* discusses the role of CHRE and suggests that it should increasingly be able to focus its efforts on harmonisation of the standards and processes of the regulators rather than on the scrutiny and challenge of individual decisions.

Annex D
Recommendations of the Ayling Inquiry

No*	Para	Inquiry recommendation	Government response	
			Para	Response
1	2.30	We therefore recommend that the DH convene an expert group under the auspices of the Chief Medical Officer to develop guidance and best practice for the NHS on this subject. The group should include the NHS Confederation, the RCOG, the RCGP (and other Colleges as appropriate, such as the Royal College of Psychiatrists), the NCAA, the CRHP, the GMC and representatives of undergraduate and postgraduate medical education. The group should take advice from experience of dealing with sexualised behaviour elsewhere in the public sector such as educational services and from health care systems in other countries such as Canada.	6.4	The government has invited CHRE to lead a project involving all relevant stakeholders to develop a comprehensive suite of guidance in this area.
2	2.31	In parallel with this, we recommend that local policies within all NHS Trusts for reporting staff concerns (whistleblowing) should specifically identify sexualised behaviour as appropriate for reporting within the confidence of this procedure.	5.33	Accept: we will follow up this recommendation as part of the action described at para 5.33 of this response.
3	2.34	We therefore recommend that accredited training should be provided for all PALS officers in this potential aspect of their work, and that SHAs should require confirmation from each NHS Trust in their area of the completion of such training within the next 12 months.	6.7–9	We agree the importance of training for PALS officers in handling allegations about boundary transgressions. The Department has developed a training programme for PALS and ICAS staff; this was initially delivered by the charity Witness and has now been rolled out nationally.

* The Ayling Inquiry did not number its recommendations; these numbers are added to facilitate cross-referencing

No*	Para	Inquiry recommendation	Government response	
			Para	Response
4	2.36	We therefore recommend that the Modernisation Agency develop a model of best practice for access to PALS especially in primary care] and, if appropriate for them so to do, the patients' forums could monitor the effectiveness of service provision against this model. The implementation of this model and associated performance measures should be a formal component of CHAI's reviews of PCTs.		The Government agrees the importance of ensuring that patients who wish to raise concerns about the quality of care they have received from the NHS are aware of the PALS services and can readily access them. The Department of Health has drawn up national standards for the work of PALS and SHAs are responsible for monitoring the quality of the services offered against these standards. In addition, the Department has commissioned an independent evaluation of the impact of PALS, conducted by the University of West England, which is due to be completed later this year. The role of PALS within future arrangements for handling complaints, in both health and social care, will be considered in the consultation described in chapter 5 of this response.
5	2.39	We recommend that the same training for ICAS staff in handling concerns and complaints of an intimate and sensitive nature as that we have recommended for PALS staff should be provided, and that this should form part of the service specification for ICAS. We also believe that satisfaction surveys should be built into the work of ICAS on completion of their work with each complaint so that their performance can be routinely monitored and a cycle of continuous improvement be established.	6.7–9	See above on recommendation 3. The supply of this type of training has been included in the ICAS service specification from April 2006 onwards. The Department routinely works with all ICAS providers to increase the amount of feedback gathered from clients and reviews the way this information is used to develop the service.

No*	Para	Inquiry recommendation	Government response	
			Para	Response
6	2.42	We recommend that all NHS Trusts and health care organisations such as deputising services directly employing staff should require them (and particularly part-time staff) to make a formal declaration of any other concurrent employment, not only for obvious health and safety reasons but also to ensure a record is kept of other organisations with an interest in the individual's performance. Failure to make such a declaration should be a disciplinary matter. This requirement should be appropriately adapted for PCTs to be kept informed of other professional employment undertaken by GP.	8.4	We recognise the importance of ensuring that PCTs and employers are aware of concurrent employment of healthcare professionals and have made arrangements to share information on concerns, especially where patient safety is at issue. We are considering ways of underlining this importance, for instance by imposing a statutory duty on health organisations to share information about health professionals where needed to safeguard patients.
7	2.44	We recommend that copies of any written records regarding complaints and concerns and the outcome of these which name an individual practitioner should be placed on that practitioner's personnel file, to be kept for the length of their contract with that organisation. This should be made known to the practitioner concerned.	8.3	Agreed – this will be covered in the guidance on the content of personnel files described in para 8.3 of the response.
8	2.45	We recommend that the regular reports on patient complaints and concerns made to NHS Trust Boards and other corporate governance bodies should be structured to provide an analysis not only of trends in subject matter and clinical area but also to indicate whether a named practitioner has been the subject of previous complaints.	4.10	We agree that clinical governance staff in healthcare organisations should analyse data on complaints and concerns in order to identify any "clusters" relating to individual health professionals. We would not necessarily expect the individuals to be named in reports to Trust Boards unless further investigation confirmed that there was significant cause for concern. For doctors, the local clinical governance team will also wish to discuss with the GMC affiliate.

No*	Para	Inquiry recommendation	Government response	
			Para	Response
9	2.48	We therefore recommend that PCTs should develop specific support programmes for single-handed practitioners, to be agreed with the practitioner concerned and the PCT's SHA. Such programmes should pay critical attention to managing the risks of clinical and professional isolation associated with single-handed practice. Implementation should be monitored by the SHA and form part of the regular CHAI review of the PCT.	4.42	Agreed in principle: the Department will discuss further with NHS and professional organisations what support would be appropriate.
10	2.49	Additionally, PCTs should pay particular attention to developing and supporting the independence of practice managers in single-handed practices, including the acknowledgment and resolution of potential conflicts of interest which may arise where the manager is the spouse or a close relative of the practitioner. This too should be the subject of monitoring and review by SHAs and CHAI.	4.42	As for previous recommendation.
11	2.58	We recommend that no family member or friend of a patient should be expected to undertake any formal chaperoning role. The presence of a chaperone during a clinical examination and treatment must be the clearly expressed choice of a patient. Chaperoning should not be undertaken by other than trained staff: the use of untrained administrative staff as chaperones in a GP surgery, for example, is not acceptable. However the patient must have the right to decline any chaperone offered if they so wish.	6.10	Agreed. Guidance on chaperoning policies for primary care organisations, covering these points, was issued in June 2005. We will discuss with NHS Employers whether specific guidance for secondary care providers is needed.

No*	Para	Inquiry recommendation	Government response	
			Para	Response
12	2.59	Beyond these immediate and practical points, there is a need for each NHS Trust to determine its chaperoning policy, make this explicit to patients and resource it accordingly. This must include accredited training for the role and an identified managerial lead with responsibility for the implementation of the policy. We recognise that for primary care, developing and resourcing a chaperoning policy will have to take into account issues such as one-to-one consultations in the patient's home and the capacity of individual practices to meet the requirements of the agreed policy.	6.10	As for previous recommendation.
13	2.60	Finally, reported breaches of the chaperoning policy should be formally investigated through each Trust's risk management and clinical governance arrangements and treated, if determined as deliberate, as a disciplinary matter.	6.11	Agreed: the government will ask CHRE to draw this recommendation to the attention of all healthcare organisations as part of the suite of guidance described at para 6.4 of the response.
14	2.63	We therefore recommend that LMCs clarify their role in relation to supporting GPs to make it explicit that acting on the receipt of information about a GP which indicates patient safety is being compromised is not part of their role, and ensure that this is embedded in professional guidance from the GMC and medical defence organisations.	5.35	The Government agrees that PCTs should have an overview of all concerns raised about the conduct of performance of health professionals working under contract for them and should take the final decision on whether any further action is needed. The Government will consult further with stakeholders and issue further guidance or amend the regulations as needed.

No*	Para	Inquiry recommendation	Government response	
			Para	Response
15	2.64	We further recommend that if LMCs are the recipient of concerns about a practitioner's clinical conduct or performance, this information should be immediately passed on to the relevant PCT or professional regulatory body for appropriate investigation. This should be made known to their constituents. We believe that not doing this would leave professional members and staff of a LMC in the potential position of having failed to meet their own professional obligations.	5.35	As for previous recommendation.
16	2.71	There should be set out in a Memorandum of Understanding (such as exists between the GMC and the NCAA) between the NHS, professional regulatory bodies such as the GMC and the CPS a clear agreement as to the responsibilities of each organisation in the investigation of potential criminal activity by health care professionals. This should then be promulgated to the NHS and built into the guidance suggested below.	4.22–23	Advice relating to investigations of potential criminal activity has recently been issued in the form of a Memorandum of Understanding between the Police, the Health and Safety Executive and the NHS. There is a similar MOU between the GMC, NMC and the Police. Guidance on the thresholds at which issues of professional competence or conduct should be referred to the professional regulators will be developed by CHRE as described at para 4.17 of *Trust, assurance and safety*.
17	2.72	We therefore recommend that SHAs work together with the Department of Health to produce guidance for PCTs and other NHS Trusts in handling such incidents [ie incidents involving potentially criminal activity], particularly since the latest reorganisation of the NHS has created a large number of relatively inexperienced PCTs with responsibility for GP contracts.	4.24, 4.12	Agreed – see previous recommendation. In addition, the Department will issue guidance covering all aspects of investigation by healthcare organisations after consultation with stakeholders.
18	2.73	We further recommend that part of the guidance we have suggested SHAs and the Department of Health develop for the NHS should specifically address a patients communications strategy and the involvement of local victim support services.	4.12	Agreed – we will ensure that this is covered in the guidance referred to in relation to the previous recommendation.

Annex E
Recommendations of the Neale Inquiry

No	Inquiry recommendation	Government response	
		Para	**Response**
1	That the Secretary of State for Health should consider setting up a new body, or expanding the power of an existing body such as the Council for Regulation of Healthcare Professionals to take an overarching view of all aspects of the rules governing the appointment and employment of doctors. This body should have necessary powers of investigation in the wider interests of patient safety, ensuring a robust and consistent approach to individual concerns that may arise in the future.	3.6	This already falls within the remit of NHS Employers, a part of the NHS Confederation.
2	Security of tenure for NHS Consultants with a Protective appeal procedure to the Secretary of Sate should be abolished	3.11	The "para 190" right of appeal to the Secretary of State was abolished in 2005. Consultants now come under the same disciplinary arrangements for misconduct as other members of staff.
3	The contents of the model declaration forms referred to in HSC2002/08 should be made mandatory in the NHS	3.8	HSC2002/08 has been superseded by more recent guidance. We will consider how the new regulatory framework can best be used to promote adoption of best practice in relation to these model declaration forms.
4	For all doctor appointments made directly from overseas, regardless of where they qualified, employing authorities should check with the issuing body the recommended applicant's primary and postgraduate qualifications and confirm fitness to practise.	3.9	The Government considers that it is for professional regulators to check the primary qualification of healthcare professionals appointed from overseas. The Government agrees that NHS organisations should check other postgraduate qualifications and will ask NHS Employers to ensure this is reflected in guidance.

No	Inquiry recommendation	Government response	
		Para	Response
5a	All references by employing authorities should specify the areas they require to be addressed by the referee.	3.10	Agreed – this is already good practice, but the Department will ask NHS Employers to ensure it is explicitly reflected in guidance.
5b	No agreement should ever be entered into to provide a reference, which in anyway negates the view that the interests and safety of the patient are paramount.	3.10	Agreed – the Government has asked CHRE to ensure that all professional regulators give guidance on the ethical responsibilities of referees and will draw this recommendation to their attention. The GMC's guidance *Good medical practice* already includes provision to this effect.
6	Only a fully completed standard application form with room for additional information should be acceptable. Amended, substituted or adapted forms should not be used for any reason.		As for recommendation 5a.
7	Clear roles should be established for all those on an interview panel and full note of proceedings should be taken and retained.	3.7	As for recommendation 5a.
8	All previous contacts between applicant and interviewers should be disclosed and recorded.	3.7	As for recommendation 5a.
9	Any undisclosed championing of applicants should be disclosed and recorded.	3.7	As for recommendation 5a.
10	The application form should contain a declaration that all information is correct to the best of the applicant's knowledge and belief and any matter, professional or personal unresolved or pending that might undermine the applicant's standing, or cause embarrassment to the NHS, should be declared by a confidential side letter to the chairman. The penalty for failure to disclose such information should be summary dismissal.	3.7	As for recommendation 5a.
11	The NHS should give consideration to instruct employers to include a condition that clinical employees must declare any police cautions or convictions to the employer as they arise after the commencement of their employment.	3.12	Current guidance from NHS Employers advises all NHS employers to include such a condition in contracts of employment. All health professionals are in addition under an ethical obligation to report cautions and convictions to their professional regulator.

No	Inquiry recommendation	Government response	
		Para	Response
12	The Panel Chairman should be responsible for ensuring that referees are contacted by telephone and content of the references should be confirmed at or around the time of appointment.	3.10	As for recommendation 5a.
13	The police check should include convictions, cautions and entries on the sex offenders Register.	3.13	Since February 2005 it has been mandatory for all NHS employers to arrange for checks at the Criminal Records Bureau (CRB) for all relevant NHS staff. The standard disclosure from the CRB shows current and spent convictions, cautions, reprimands and warnings held on the Police National Computer.
14	Employing authorities/medical colleagues should not give a reference which is capable of being misleading by omission.	3.10	See above on recommendations 5a and 5b.
15	Patients should receive copies of letters sent to and from their general practitioners and in the template of the letter sent to all patients, the doctor should confirm, "I have discussed the condition and treatment with the patient."	8.20–21	DH issued guidance on implementing the initiative "Copying letters to patients" in 2003. This includes suggested templates setting out the information that can be included in letters, including items like diagnosis, management recommendations and the results of investigations as well information given to patients. Patients should be asked whether they wish to receive copies of letters and their decision should be recorded in local systems. The underlying principle is that the written information to patients should reinforce the information they have already been given in consultations, which will naturally include the patient's condition and the recommended treatment for which they are being referred.

No	Inquiry recommendation	Government response	
		Para	Response
16	In the patient's copy of the discharge letter the doctor should complete as appropriate, that, "the procedure went to plan/had the following complications... This has/has not been discussed with the patient".	8.20–21	See comment on previous recommendation. It would be poor clinical practice to give patients information in writing which had not previously been discussed face to face. Professional guidance from the GMC and from the medical defence organisations encourages doctors to be open with their patients about complications or adverse events, but the level of detail of the information to be disclosed must be ultimately for the professional judgement of the clinician and we would not want to be prescriptive in this sensitive area.
17	If a consultant has not performed a procedure or part of a procedure himself he should legibly identify who did and whether it was under supervision. Patients should know who operated on them.	8.20–21	See on previous recommendation.
18	Clear procedures should be set up so that the patient may give consent for a nominated third party to act as their advocate in raising concerns if they are unable to do so.		Accept – this power already exists in the complaints regulations. As part of the review of the complaints procedures we will ensure that patients and carers are made aware of the position.
19	Doctors should spend time observing the Patient Advocacy and Liaison Service (PALS) process and be familiar with the process.		This is already common practice; many PALS staff already provide input to induction and other training programes for clinical staff.
20	All PALS appointees should be of middle/senior grade.		NHS Employers will shortly be publishing five new national core job descriptions/gradings, ranging from PALS officer through to a senior management role. This will enable Trusts to understand better the responsibilities of each role and to support the development of the service nationwide.

No	Inquiry recommendation	Government response	
		Para	**Response**
21	Unified and centralised training should be provided for all PALS officers.		The Department of Health sets national standards for PALS training, but SHAs also have an important role in ensuring that local health communities carry out an appropriate analysis of specific training needs and provide the training needed. Centralised training has been arranged on occasions, in response to particular national needs, but this is not the norm.
22	Complaints handling should be aligned to quality management and patient services rather than claims management.	4.13–14	Accept. The government fully agrees that complaints handling should be regarded as an integral part of clinical governance and that complaints should be seen as a vital source of information for improving the quality of services and identifying any potentially unsafe practice. The government will consider with stakeholders how existing statutory responsibilities can be strengthened.
23	The head of the unit dealing with complaints should be an appropriately trained manager.	5.12–13	The Department agrees that complaints handlers in PCTs or hospital trusts should be appointed at a sufficiently senior level and with appropriate training, and that they should have direct access to the member of the executive board with overall responsibility for clinical governance issues.
24	Complaints handling training should be mandatory for all levels of clinical, nursing and administrative staff.		The Government agrees that all front line NHS staff need to have an awareness of local complaints handling processes so that complaints, wherever they are received in the organisation, are swiftly transferred to the complaints handling team. We will address the implications for training and induction processes in the review of the complaints system described in chapter 5 of this response.

No	Inquiry recommendation	Government response	
		Para	Response
25	The National Patient Safety Agency should take the lead in developing adverse event reporting systems. Data taken from complaints should be integrated with and/or read alongside other data from such sources as confidential reports on near misses, patient satisfaction surveys and clinical and medical audit.	4.10, 8.3, 8.9–10	The Government agrees that it is vital for local information systems to be able to integrate information from different sources such as complaints, clinical audit, patient satisfaction surveys and adverse incident reports, in order to identify clusters of indicators which might point to poor professional performance or systems failures. Some PCTs have developed impressive "practice profile" systems of this kind. At present the NPSA's core role is to collect patient safety incident data from local reporting systems and other sources through the National Reporting and Learning System and the Patient Safety Observatory The Observatory analyses these incident data alongside other national level data relevant to safety, eg clinical negligence claims from the NHS Litigation Authority. In the light of the recent report *Safety First* the Department of Health and NPSA are reviewing the future role of NPSA and of local patient safety action teams in encouraging the development of integrated local systems.
26	Complaints statistics should be included in the Profiles of Trusts and used by CHAI (now referred to as the Healthcare Commission) in routine audit procedures.		This is already the case.
27	Statutory provision should be made to encourage the reporting of adverse events.	5.38	The government agrees the importance of encouraging health professionals to report any concerns about the safety of services but considers that this is better promoted by professional ethical guidance rather than through statutory provision. A proposed "duty of candour" was rejected by Parliament during debate on the 2006 NHS Redress Act.

Annex F
Recommendations of the Kerr/Haslam Inquiry

No*	Page no	Inquiry recommendation	Government response	
			Para	**Comment**
1		One of the referees in any job application should be the consultant who conducts the applicant's appraisal, their Clinical Director, or their Medical Director.	3.10	The Government will invite NHS Employers to reflect this principle in updated guidance to employers.
2	35	Procedures and policies should be put in place, within twelve months of the publication of this Report, to ensure that all NHS organisations are aware of the therapies being undertaken by all staff, particularly those where patients believe clinical governance committees should be aware of them and making decisions about their use.	4.43	The Government agrees that clinical governance committees should be aware of all "new and unorthodox treatments" in use within the healthcare organisation, whether in mental health or in other sectors. The Department of Health will shortly be issuing revised guidance to clinical governance committees on the steps needed to ensure patient safety in adopting innovative treatments.
3	35	Within mental health services no member of the health care team should be permitted to use or pursue new or unorthodox treatments without discussion and approval by the team (such approval to be recorded in writing).	4.43	See previous recommendation. Where care is delivered on a team basis, clinical governance committees will wish to assure themselves that proposals to use new therapies are supported by the consensus view of the team.
4	24	In relation to such identified "new or unorthodox treatments", patients should be given written explanations of the treatments, and why their use is appropriate.	4.43, 8.17	See recommendation 2. The Government agrees that patients need appropriate information to give informed consent to any treatment and that this is particularly important for new or unorthodox treatments. The Department will cover these aspects in the guidance referred to above.

* The Kerr/Haslam Inquiry did not number its recommendations; these numbers are added to facilitate cross-referencing.

No*	Page no	Inquiry recommendation	Government response	
			Para	**Comment**
5	24	The full range of physical, psychological and complementary therapies used by mental health professionals should be recorded and discussed through appraisal/job plans. Trusts should have a clear evidence base and protocols for guiding the use of these treatments.		See recommendation 2. Where a mental health professional is using a new or unorthodox therapy we would expect that to be discussed at appraisal, and will ensure that this principle is covered in the guidance referred to above. Existing guidance on appraisal for both hospital consultants and GPs already specifies that the appraisal should cover all clinical aspects of the doctor's work.
6	25	The NHS should reconsider whether or not statutory regulation should be extended to cover hypnotherapy.		Hypnotherapy is not a discrete profession in its own right but a technique which is used by a variety of disciplines. The Government is intending to introduce statutory regulation for some of the better established psychological disciplines including applied psychologists, psychotherapists and other psychological therapists. See chapter 7 of *Trust, assurance and safety* for further discussion of the approach to regulation of emerging professions.
7	25	When appointments to the NHS are considered, references should be obtained from the three most recent employers and those references should be properly checked.	3.10	The government agrees that panel chairmen should always be alert to the possibility of misleading references, including references from a much earlier part of the candidate's career, and will ask NHS Employers to consider how this principle could be reflected in updated guidance.

No*	Page no	Inquiry recommendation	Government response	
			Para	**Comment**
8	25	The Department of Health should develop and publish a specific policy, with practical guidance on implementation, to guide NHS managers in their handling of allegations or disclosure of sexualised behaviour. The policy should address the various issues and difficulties set out above and include examples of good practice, as well as the extended range of options for action that could be applied; where advice and assistance can readily be provided; guidance on record-making and keeping. The guidance should also include a range of preventative measures (for example, specific accessible information for patients on what they should and should not expect in consultations, and who they can speak to for confidential advice and assistance).	6.6	The Department of Health accepts these recommendations and is asking CHRE to progress them as part of the project referred to in para 6.4 of this response.
9	26	In relation to disclosures of alleged abuse, voluntary advocacy and advice services (independent of the NHS) should be supported by central public funding to offer advice and assistance to patients and former patients (particularly those who are mentally unwell, or who are otherwise vulnerable).	6.7–9	All ICAS advocates have received mental health awareness training and an increasing number across the country have received specialist training in order to be able to support clients with allegations of abuse.
10	26	All Trusts should develop, within their Code of Behaviour , guidance to reduce the likelihood of sexualised behaviour, that is incorporated into the contracts of employment of those staff, or contracts of engagement for all other persons providing mental health services within the NHS.	6.4	The CHRE project described at para 6.4 of this response will develop guidance both for professionals and for healthcare organisations on how to minimise the risk of boundary violations in all therapeutic situations, including mental health services.

No*	Page no	Inquiry recommendation	Government response	
			Para	Comment
11	26	Regarding mental health services, the NHS should review the cut-off period for registering a complaint, as well as the criteria for initiating an investigation of an old complaint and the procedures to be applied.		The Government agrees in principle that the cut-off period and the criteria for investigating older complaints should be reviewed (in all disciplines, not just in mental health), provided that it is still possible to investigate fairly. This will be covered in the review of the complaints procedure described in chapter 5 of this response.
12	26	Protocols should be established to ensure that psychiatric patients who raise concerns or complaints in relation to allegations of abuse are not treated in ways which are less favourable than the treatment advised for vulnerable or intimidated witnesses within the framework of "Achieving Best Evidence" (Action For Justice, 2002). Such psychiatric patients should be treated with care, consideration and integrity.		Accept – again this should apply to all disciplines and not just in mental health. We will pick this up in the review of the complaints procedure described in chapter 5 of this response.
13	26	Because medical procedures that require benzodiazepines to be given intravenously (e.g. oral endoscopy and induction of anaesthesia) are potentially high risk in terms of false sexual fantasies and allegations, these should always be chaperoned (see Chapter 31, Chaperones).	6.10	Accepted in principle, although intravenous benzodiazepines may sometimes be needed in emergencies when a chaperone may not be available. We will cover this in any further updates of the general NHS guidance on chaperones – see para 6.10 of this response.
14	26	Trusts' confidentiality policies should include a section on disclosure within therapeutic interactions in psychiatric practice and should be supported by inter-agency information-sharing policies to be used in all cases of patient abuse.	7.6	Accept in principle; the Department of Health is developing guidance in this area and hopes to issue it in the spring.

No*	Page no	Inquiry recommendation	Government response	
			Para	Comment
15	27	Dedicated staff should be properly trained to carry out the investigations. This relates closely to the recommendations we make at the end of Chapter 33 regarding investigations generally.	4.15, 5.10	Accept. Existing standards already require healthcare organisations to operate effective systems for handling complaints. As part of the review of the health and social care complaints system described in chapter 5 of this response, the Department of Health will seek views on how these standards could be strengthened.
16	27	The Secretary of State, within 12 months of the publication of this Report, should commission and publish guidance and issue advice and instruction (preferably in consultation with the professional regulatory bodies and healthcare Colleges) as to the meaning and limitations of patient confidentiality in mental health settings. Such guidance should be kept under regular review.	7.6	See above on recommendation 14.
17	27	The NHS should convene an expert group to consider what boundaries need to be set between patients and mental health staff who have been in long-term therapeutic relationships, and how those boundaries are to be respected in terms of guidelines for the behaviour of health service professionals, and the provision of safeguards for patients.	6.4	Accept. This will be covered in the CHRE project described in chapter 6 of this response.
18	27	Detailed, and readily accessible, guidance should be developed for medical professionals. The guidance should be framed in terms which address conduct which will not be tolerated and which is likely to lead to disciplinary action. Such guidance, if not provided at a professional regulatory level, should be supplemented by the NHS at an employment level.	6.4	As above.

No*	Page no	Inquiry recommendation	Government response	
			Para	Comment
19	27	Policies should be developed that enable health workers to feel able to disclose feelings of sexual attraction at the earliest stage possible without the automatic risk of disciplinary proceedings. Colleagues must also feel able to discuss openly and report concerns about the development of attraction/overly familiar relationships with patients. These policies should include all grade levels, including consultant.	6.4	As above.
20	27	The Secretary of State, within 12 months of the publication of this Report, should convene an expert group to develop guidance and best practice for the NHS on boundary setting, boundary transgression, sexualised behaviour, and all forms of abuse of patients, in the mental health services.	6.4	As above.
21	28	The terms of reference of the expert group should not be restricted to sexualised behaviour between psychiatrists (or other mental healthcare professionals) and current patients, but should also address former patients.	6.4	As above.
22	28	There should be detailed research carried out and published by the Department of Health to show the prevalence of sexual assaults, sexual contact, or other sexualised behaviour, between doctors and existing and/or former patients – particularly in the field of mental health.	6.5	The CHRE project described above will review current research on the profile of people perpetrating boundary violations. In the light of this review the Department of Health will consider whether to commission further comprehensive research on the prevalence of sexualised behaviour.

No*	Page no	Inquiry recommendation	Government response	
			Para	**Comment**
23	28	The Department of Health should urgently investigate and report upon the need for a co-ordinated method of mandatory data collection and mandatory recording, in relation to the area of abuse of patients by mental healthcare professionals.	6.5	The Department of Health will encourage the professional regulators to carry out a retrospective analysis of recent fitness to practice cases to determine in what proportion boundary violations have been a factor. The Department of Health will also consider whether the information received from reports of Serious Untoward Incidents could be categorised so as to allow routine analysis of this kind.
24	28	Mental health services should provide routine information to patients attending appointments on what to expect from a consultation with a mental health professional. This should apply to consultations in all settings, including home visits.	8.17–19	The Government agrees that, where a novel or unusual therapy is to be offered, patients should receive a full written explanation in advance (see above on recommendation 4). For more conventional therapies it is reasonable to expect that the referrer will have described in broad terms the likely assessment and therapeutic purpose of the consultation. Many GPs and hospital outpatient clinics will reinforce this by providing information leaflets. The Department of Health is developing an Information Accreditation Scheme which will raise the general standard of such information and help the public to find reliable sources of information. We are also testing out a set of "questions to ask" to help people, including those in disadvantaged groups, to prepare for consultations and empower them to ask appropriate questions.

No*	Page no	Inquiry recommendation	Government response	
			Para	Comment
25	28	Where physical contact forms part of the consultation, or where there is a risk of loss of consciousness, there should be should be a national policy and implementation guidelines to safeguard patients and staff and support the maintenance of appropriate boundaries.	6.4	Accept – this will be covered in the CHRE project described in chapter 6 of this response.
26	28	The NHS should review current records management practice and ensure that a robust set of systems and practices are uniformly applied across the service.		The Government agrees that clinical records should be made at or close to the time of the original consultation and that any subsequent amendments should be clearly documented. This is a key principle of *Connecting for Health*. The Department of Health will ask the professional regulators to ensure that their ethical guidance underlines the importance of accurate clinical records and makes clear that any deliberate falsification would call into question the clinician's fitness to practise.
27	28	Within 12 months of publication of this Report, the Department of Health should issue guidance as to how and where any disclosure or complaint of abuse by another healthcare professional made to a doctor or nurse should be recorded (if at all) in the patient's medical records, and elsewhere.	8.3 and 8.6	Accept in principle. The Department of Health will work with stakeholders to develop guidance on the content of the files to be held by healthcare organisations relating to the performance of individual professionals, including complaints and concerns. It would not normally be appropriate for such information to be held in the patient's clinical records and the Department will consider, as part of the wider review of the complaints system, whether further guidance is needed on this point.

No*	Page no	Inquiry recommendation	Government response	
			Para	Comment
28	29	A protocol should be produced, and guidance issued within 12 months of the publication of this Report regarding the collection, collation and retention of data in relation to concerns and complaints covering sexualised conduct by mental health professionals – including, but not restricted to: a. The name of the mental health professional; b. The details of the concern or complaint; c. The date of the alleged sexualised behaviour; d. The date of the concern or complaint; e. If investigated, by whom and with what outcome; f. If not investigated, the reason.	8.3 and 8.6	As for previous recommendation.
29	29	Consideration should be given to the retention period of such data, stating our preference (subject to the advice of the Information Commissioner, and the terms of the Human Rights Act 1998) that such data be retained for the lifetime of the mental health professional. All NHS staff should be made aware regularly that this data is collected and retained.	8.3 and 8.6	As above.
30a	29	The current regulations relating to complaints procedures should be amended to enable any person with a concern about the safety and effectiveness of the NHS to be allowed more readily to use the NHS complaints procedure.		The Government agrees that the complaints procedure should be as simple as possible for patients and their representatives to use; this is one of the key principles of the review of the complaints system described in chapter 5 of this response. For people with a generalised rather than personal concern about safety and effectiveness of the NHS a number of possible routes are available, including the PALS services.
30b	29	Further the time limit applicable from the incidents complained of and the complaint being made should be relaxed.		Accept – see on recommendation 11 above.

No*	Page no	Inquiry recommendation	Government response	
			Para	Comment
31	29	The Department of Health review the effectiveness of whistleblowing policies and initiatives within NHS-funded organisations.	5.32–37	The Government fully agrees the need to support healthcare workers who wish to raise concerns about the services in which they work or the performance of individual professionals. See chapter 5 of this response.
32	29	As a matter of some urgency the NHS should clarify the context of the positive obligation of NHS staff to inform NHS management of concerns in relation to the suspicion of the abuse of patients.	5.37	This principle is already covered in ethical guidance from the professional regulators and from NCAS. We will discuss with the professional regulatory bodies and universities how this duty can be further emphasised especially in undergraduate education.
33	30	Policies and guidance should be drawn up to clarify the obligation to investigate (certainly in the case of suspicion of the abuse of possibly vulnerable patients) without the need for a complaint from, or that identifies, a particular named patient.	4.12	The Government agrees that all concerns, from whatever source, should be fully investigated especially where there are allegations of abuse. This will be covered in the guidance referred to at para 4.12 of this response.
34	30	The NHS should, jointly with the appropriate National Standards bodies, produce a standardised complaints system to be implemented in all Trusts/ organisations providing services to NHS patients.	5.10–11	The Government agrees that the complaints system should be as far as possible integrated across health and social care. As part of the wider review discussed in chapter 5 of this response the Department of Health will consider how the current standards for complaints handling should be strengthened.
35	30	Themes and trends arising from the data of complaints, incidents, patient and carer feedback should be analysed on a regular basis. This should form part of clinical governance and used to give early warning of emerging patterns of risk behaviour, in the interests of patient safety.	4.10–12	Accept. This will be covered in the guidance referred to at para 4.12 of this response.

No*	Page no	Inquiry recommendation	Government response	
			Para	Comment
36	30	Information about the NHS complaints procedure and its relationship to other forms of regulation and clinical governance should be explained to all staff during their induction process and form a core part of continuing professional development programmes. This should include advice and training on how to deal with distressed and angry patients who want to make a complaint.	5.18–20	Accept. We will consider the best way of promoting awareness of complaints handling procedures in all NHS staff as part of the work on common standards for initial handling and rerouting of complaints (see para 5.20 of this response).
37	30	Frontline staff who receive complaints about issues which compromise patient safety – whether or not in the confines of a therapeutic disclosure – should be under an express obligation to report that matter to a complaints manager (in or beyond their own organisation) whether or not they work for the organisation named in the complaint.	5.18–20, 5.37	Accept – see on previous recommendation and also on recommendation 32.
38	30	Health and social care commissions should resource independent mental health advocacy as a priority.	6.7–9	See above on recommendation 9.
39	31	PALS and complaints staff should be actively linked into a clinical governance and information sharing network with regular access to data on performance issues drawn from such things as claims, patient satisfaction surveys, audit and peer review.	8.6, 8.7	Accept in principle. The Department of Health will discuss with stakeholders the ways in which information relating to the performance of individual professionals can be shared within and between health organisations. For doctors, information relating to substantiated concerns (eg local disciplinary action or "Recorded Concerns") will be held on the GMC Register and accessible to appropriate individuals in accredited healthcare organisations. See *Trust, assurance and safety* chapter 6.
40	31	PALS and complaints staff should have direct access to a line manager at board level and to senior medical staff and that they should be appointed at middle management level.	5.12	Accept. We will cover this point in the review of complaints procedures described in chapter 5 of this response.

No*	Page no	Inquiry recommendation	Government response	
			Para	Comment
41	31	The roles of complaints officer and PALS officer should be distinct.		As for previous recommendation.
42	31	The Department of Health should introduce permanent arrangements for the provision of independent advice for mental health patients.	7.7	Accept in principle. The majority of ICAS advocates have now had specialist training in mental health issues.
43	31	The Department of Health should be responsible for ensuring a standardised training programme for PALS and NHS complaints staff.	5.13, 5.31	Accept in principle. Training courses are already available and the Department of Health is also setting up a national network to enable complaints staff, including those in primary care, to share best practice.
44	31	Those who are given the task of responding and initiating any investigation should themselves be adequately trained, equipped with the necessary skills to carry matters forward, and of such seniority as to ensure that barriers and resistance are overcome.	4.15, 4.18, 4.34, 5.10	Accept. See previous recommendation for training of front-line complaints staff. For the more complex investigations or those involving more serious allegations front-line NHS organisations may wish to call on additional resources such as the multi-PCT agencies discussed at para 4.34 of this response.
45	31	The revised regulations should require that all formal complaints should be directed to designated complaints managers in PCTs and NHS Trusts.	5.20, 5.25–26	The Department of Health will develop standards to ensure that complaints, wherever they are initially received, are speedily routed to the most appropriate organisation (and to the complaints manager in that organisation). See further on recommendation 36 above. In primary medical care, we propose subject to consultation to allow patients or their representative to make complaints directly to the PCT rather than to the GP practice.
46	31	Formal complaints should be interpreted as any matter which the complainants would like to be treated as formal.	5.8, 5.10	Accept. This is already the formal position, but we will consider in the wider review of the complaints system how to promote greater awareness.

No*	Page no	Inquiry recommendation	Government response	
			Para	Comment
47	31	Current regulations should be amended to ensure that it is the duty of complaints officers to investigate complaints in a speedy, efficient and effective manner.	5.10, 4.13–14	Accept in principle. However, the Government considers that it is more important to ensure that the handling of complaints achieves desirable outcomes (eg protection of patient safety) than to meet rigid targets for response times. These points will be covered in the work on standards for complaints handling described in para 5.10 of this response; see also paras 4.13–14 on the need for robust investigation of complaints.
48	31	Current regulations should be amended to require complaints managers to consider the implications for clinical governance and patient safety of all complaints received. Where a clinical governance issue arises this should be reported to their line manager and to the board.	5.8, 5.10	Accept in principle. This will be covered in the wider review of complaints handling, in particular the proposed strengthening of the national standards for complaints handling.
49	32	Current regulations should be amended, and suitable guidance prepared, to allow and ensure that complaints managers consider the reference of any complaint received which, if true, would disclose the commission of a crime, to the local police force.	4.22	Accept in principle. A recent Memorandum of Understanding between the NHS, ACPO and HSE required NHS investigators to liaise with the police and discuss handling in all cases involving potential criminal behaviour.
50	32	Current regulations should be amended to require complaints managers to take statements from all those staff involved in the investigation of the complaint.	5.10	As for recommendation 48.
51	32	Guidance issued under the regulations should clarify what constitutes a full and rigorous investigation, most notably that complaints officers be placed under a duty to raise additional issues for investigation.	5.10	As for recommendation 48.

No*	Page no	Inquiry recommendation	Government response	
			Para	Comment
52	32	All NHS staff should be placed under an obligation to co-operate with investigations carried out by complaints managers.		Accepted. All NHS employed staff are required to comply with the reasonable requests of their employer and are expected to comply with local procedures for the investigation of complaints, critical incidents or concerns about employees. Similarly in primary care, contractors have a contractual obligation to cooperate with investigations undertaken by the PCT, Healthcare Commission or other bodies. The Department will discuss with stakeholders how these duties could be reinforced through ethical guidance from the professional regulators.
53	32	Where possible, the NHS should give clear advice and guidance on employment protocols following allegations of abuse.	6.6	Accepted. The Department of Health will invite CHRE to develop guidance as part of the project referred to in para 6.4 of this response.
54	32	Chief Executives acting on the advice of their complaints managers should be given the authority to refer a complaint to the Healthcare Commission for further consideration.	4.19	The government is not convinced that front-line healthcare organisations should have an automatic right to refer complex complaints to the Healthcare Commission. However where initial investigation suggests some deeper structural problems in the organisation NHS bodies may wish to alert the Commission, which may in turn decide to investigate those incidents which meet its investigation criteria.
55	32	Complainants should be allowed to pursue litigation at the same time as a complaint is being investigated.	4.24	Accepted. We will give further guidance as part of the guidance referred to at para 4.12 of this response.

No*	Page no	Inquiry recommendation	Government response	
			Para	Comment
56	32	The Department of Health should convene a working party to consider what information it is necessary to record about complaints in order for them to be of use in clinical governance and the circumstances and form in which it is appropriate to record suspicions.	8.6	Agree in principle. The Department will develop guidance for the NHS as part of the wider guidance on the content of files on individual professionals described in para 8.6 of this response.
57	32	In line with the recommendations of the Shipman Inquiry, a centralised database [should] be set up which is capable of recording a range of information about the performance of individual doctors.	8.7	Agree in principle. For doctors, the GMC register will act as the central depository of information on the registration status of doctors, together with any related information including disciplinary action by employers and alert notices. See *Trust, assurance, safety* chapter 6.
58	33	Regulatory bodies (with responsibility for the regulation and discipline of psychiatrists and other mental healthcare professionals) and the Department of Health should be under a clear duty, in the public interest, to share information about disciplinary investigations or other related proceedings. This duty should extend to information known to the regulatory bodies and the Department of Health relating to disciplinary investigations and related proceedings, even if conducted outside the United Kingdom. Consideration should be given to the collection and retention of all information relevant to patient safety, including unsubstantiated complaints, unproven allegations and informal concerns.	8.6–7	Accept. The Department will discuss with stakeholders the concept of a "duty of collaboration" which would require healthcare organisations (including professional regulators) to share information about individual professionals where needed to protect patient safety. The Medical Act already requires the GMC to disclose information to DH and employers at the point at which they begin to investigate a case, and this is now routine practice.
59a	33	The Department of Health should clearly state what information can be included in relation to electronic staff records relating to complaints, proven/ unproven incidents, disciplinary investigations and findings. Such a record should be established in standard form and, once established, should move with the individual to reduce the risk of staff evading detection of past misdemeanours.	8.6	Accept – see on recommendation 56 above.

No*	Page no	Inquiry recommendation	Government response	
			Para	Comment
59b	33	The Department of Health should consider whether or not, and if so how and in what circumstances, any such information should be transferable between the NHS and the private sector.	8.6	Accept. This will be covered in the discussion on information sharing described in relation to recommendation 58 above.
60	33	The Department of Health in association with NIMHE and the Royal College of Psychiatrists should publish guidance in relation to clinical supervision of consultant and career grade psychiatrists.	7.8	The government does not accept that the risks associated with autonomous clinical practice are different in kind for psychiatry as compared to other clinical disciplines. The general safeguards described in this document and in *Trust, assurance and safety* should be sufficient to ensure that any poor practice or deliberate abuse is rapidly identified and dealt with, in psychiatry as in other disciplines.
61	33	Any deviation from acceptable practice [in applying the principles of the new disciplinary framework for doctors] in mental health services should be identified by the relevant statutory regulatory body and, where appropriate, by Monitor, and a standard, fair and transparent set of rules governing conduct of all mental health NHS staff in all NHS bodies and Foundation Trusts be quickly established.	7.9	Trust Boards have the primary responsibility of ensuring that good practice in relation to the new disciplinary framework for doctors is applied throughout the trust. Where the Healthcare Commission identify any significant deviations, we would expect them to draw this to the attention of the Trust board and to Monitor or the SHA as appropriate. If necessary, further regulatory action might follow.
62	34	The Secretary of State should invite the CRHE to consider (with a grant of additional powers if necessary), in relation to the regulation of healthcare professionals, the application of common standards, practices and procedures so that patient safety can more effectively be protected.		CHRE's role already includes the development of common standards and processes across the health professional regulators. This is likely to be an increasingly important part of their activities. See chapter 1 of *Trust, assurance and safety*.

No*	Page no	Inquiry recommendation	Government response	
			Para	Comment
63	34	Within 12 months of the publication of this Report the Department of Health should develop and publish national advice and guidance to Primary and Secondary Health Care Trusts addressing the [action to be taken by staff on the] disclosure of sexual, or other, abuse by patients or other service users, with particular emphasis on users of mental health services.	6.6	This will be covered in the guidance described in relation to recommendation 8 above.
64	34	The GP curriculum should be reviewed to ensure that sufficient focus is given to the needs, treatment and care of patients experiencing mental health problems and illnesses and that all GPs should have some exposure to psychiatry.	7.10	The Department is sympathetic to these recommendations and will discuss them with professional and educational interests.
65	34	Mental health issues should be part of the NMC Foundation Year 2.	7.10	As for previous recommendation.
66	34	Early consideration should be given to extending the remit of the NCAS to cover other healthcare professionals, particularly those providing care and treatment in mental health services.	4.17	The Department and NCAS are now considering, in the light of the general guidance recently drawn up by a multi-professional working party, the possible extension of the remit of NCAS to other professions.
67	34	The NHS should review the curriculum content – at all education and training levels – to ensure that medical practitioners are able to undertake appropriate cross-sector working (including within NHS i.e. primary/ secondary boundary) as part of their practice.	7.10	Accepted. The need for cross-boundary working is already recognised as an increasingly important part of training and CPD but will consider with educational and professional interests what more could be done.
68a	34	Those responsible for developing the curricula for education programmes of healthcare professionals should ensure that 1) information about and discussion of the ethical responsibilities of healthcare professionals to bring poor performance to light is given due weight.	5.37	Accepted: we will discuss with the professional regulatory bodies and universities how this duty can be further emphasised especially in undergraduate education.

No*	Page no	Inquiry recommendation	Government response	
			Para	Comment
68b	35	Those responsible for developing the curricula for education programmes of healthcare professionals should ensure that ... 2) students are made aware of: forms of regulation and clinical governance operating in the NHS and the ethos which underpins them; the relationship between the different systems; and how they can be accessed.		Accepted in principle, although educational programmes of this kind may have more impact as part of postgraduate education or continuous professional development, when health professionals are already coming into regular contact with local clinical governance systems (see above on recommendation 36 with specific reference to complaints). We will discuss further with educational and NHS interests.
69	35	Professional training includes: compulsory education and training on the maintenance of professional boundaries, awareness of boundary transgressions, sexualised behaviour as unethical conduct, response to expressions of concerns and complaints, complaints' systems, what to do if a complaint is made but the person making the complaint declines to take an active part in a formal complaint, as well as the requirements of, and limitations on, patient confidentiality.	6.4	Accepted: this will be covered in the professional guidance developed in the CHRE project described above.
70	35	The NHS should adopt and reinforce the recommendations in the Manzoor Report and in Making Amends, that there should be a duty of candour imposed on, and accepted by, NHS staff. This duty would mean that there is a responsibility to be proactively informative with patients and with their relatives and carers.		Members of the medical, nursing and midwifery professions are already under a professional obligation to inform patients when things go wrong during treatment. The Government made clear in debates on the NHS Redress Act why it did not consider it appropriate to impose a statutory duty on top of these professional obligations, and the Shipman Inquiry came to a similar conclusion in their Fifth Report. We will discuss with the CHRE and the other regulators whether a similar approach could be adopted for the other health professions.

No*	Page no	Inquiry recommendation	Government response	
			Para	Comment
71	35	In relation to private inquiries for witnesses who make statements, and/ or who give oral evidence, legal safeguards should be introduced to grant them immunity from action in relation to their evidence (whether fact or opinion), in the absence of malice.		Accepted and implemented as section 37 of the Inquiries Act 2005.
72	35	If not already appointed, a multidisciplinary committee should be established to collate, consider and report on the recommendations made in this Report, in the Shipman Report, the Neale Report, the Ayling Report, and the Peter Green Report, insofar as those reports, and the recommendations made in them relate to the common theme of handling concerns and complaints, and to patient protection.	9.13	Accepted. We will establish a multi-disciplinary national advisory group, with representation from all key stakeholders, to advise the Department on the implementation of the action programme set out in this response and in *Trust, assurance and safety*.
73	36	All Strategic Health Authorities should set up a manned telephone Helpline (perhaps called a 'PatientLine'), where anonymised (or identified) concerns could be received and processed. Any information received through the Helpline should be logged and received in confidence (unless there is express identification of the caller), and if there is sufficient information disclosed, should be discussed with the relevant NHS Trust or PCT. Consideration should be given as to how this information could best be collated either regionally or nationally.	5.32, 5.35	The Government believes that staff with concerns over patient safety issues should be invited in the first instance to share their concerns in confidence with local management. We recognise however that there are situations (not just in primary care) in which staff feel unable to raise their concerns with the organisation in which they work. In these circumstances, the PCT or SHA may have a role to play; we will explore this in more detail with stakeholders.

No*	Page no	Inquiry recommendation	Government response	
			Para	**Comment**
74	36	The Mental Health Trusts, together with the Primary Care Trusts, should draw up and distribute patient information leaflets, so that patients referred by their General Practitioners to the care of a consultant psychiatrist can better understand what to expect, and the circumstances if any in which the patient can expect to receive any physical examination or treatment from the psychiatrist. This leaflet information should include the following topics: a. when the patient can expect a physical examination by the psychiatrist; b. a description of boundaries, and what is and what is not acceptable behaviour by the psychiatrist; c. what the patient is likely to expect in the course of talking therapies (for example, questions and inquiries which some may consider too intrusive and intimate); d. what, if anything, is expected of the patient; e. the availability of trained chaperones and, if installed, the use of virtual chaperones f. the contact details of the person to whom they may turn in confidence to discuss any issue that may give them concern before, during and after treatment.		See above on recommendation 24.

Printed in the UK for The Stationery Office Limited
on behalf of the Controller of Her Majesty's Stationery Office
ID5501495 02/07
Printed on Paper containing 75% fibre content minimum.